EURYTHMY AS VISIBLE SPEECH

Man is a form proceeding out of movement. Eurythmy is a continuation of divine movement, of the divine form in man. By means of Eurythmy man approaches nearer the divine than he otherwise could.

EURYTHMY AS VISIBLE SPEECH

RUDOLF STEINER

FIFTEEN LECTURES GIVEN AT
Dornach, Switzerland, 24th June to 12th July, 1924

TRANSLATED BY VERA AND JUDY COMPTON-BURNETT

RUDOLF STEINER PRESS
LONDON

First Published 1931
Reprinted 1944
Revised edition 1956 from the second German edition
edited by I. de Jaager, 1955
Reprinted 1984

Translated and revised by Vera and Judy Compton-Burnett from
shorthand reports unrevised by the lecturer. The original
German text is published in the Complete Edition of the works
of Rudolf Steiner entitled, *Eurythmie als sichtbare Sprache* (No.
279 in the Bibliographical Survey 1961). This English edition is
published in agreement with the Rudolf Steiner Nachlassverwal-
tung, Dornach, Switzerland.

Illustrations by Assja Turgeniff from the Blackboard Sketches
by Rudolf Steiner.

Printed and bound at
The Camelot Press Ltd, Southampton

CONTENTS

ABOUT THE TRANSCRIPTS OF LECTURES

Extract from *Rudolf Steiner, An Autobiography*, Chapter 35, pp. 386–388, 2nd Edition 1980, Steinerbooks, New York.

'The results of my anthroposophical work are, first, the books available to the general public; secondly, a great number of lecture-courses, originally regarded as private publications and sold only to members of the Theosophical (later Anthroposophical) Society. The courses consist of more or less accurate notes taken at my lectures, which for lack of time I have not been able to correct. I would have preferred the spoken word to remain the spoken word. But the members wished to have the courses printed for private circulation. Thus they came into existence. Had I been able to correct them the restriction *for members only* would have been unnecessary from the beginning. As it is, the restriction was dropped more than a year ago.

In my autobiography it is especially necessary to say a word about how my books for the general public on the one hand, and the privately printed courses on the other, belong within what I elaborate as Anthroposophy.

Someone who wishes to trace my inner struggle and effort to present Anthroposophy in a way that is suitable for present-day consciousness must do so through the writings published for general distribution. In these I define my position in relation to the philosophical striving of the present. They contain what to my *spiritual sight* became ever more clearly defined, the edifice of Anthroposophy—certainly incomplete in many ways.

But another requirement arose, different from that of elaborating Anthroposophy and devoting myself solely to problems connected with imparting facts directly from the spiritual world to the general cultural life of today: the requirement of meeting fully the inner need and spiritual longing of the members.

Especially strong were the requests to have light thrown by Anthroposophy upon the Gospels and the Bible in general. The members wished to have courses of lectures on these revelations bestowed upon mankind.

In meeting this need through private lecture courses, another factor arose: at these lectures only members were present. They were familiar with basic content of Anthroposophy. I could address them as people advanced in anthroposophical knowledge. The approach I adopted in these lectures was not at all suitable for the written works intended primarily for the general public.

In these private circles I could formulate what I had to say in a way I should have been *obliged* to modify had it been planned initially for the general public.

Thus the public and the private publications are in fact two quite different things, built upon different foundations. The public writings are the direct result of my inner struggles and labours, whereas the privately printed material includes the inner struggle and labour of the members. I listened to the inner needs of the members, and my living experience of this determined the form of the lectures.

However, nothing was ever said that was not solely the result of my direct experience of the growing content of Anthroposophy. There was never any question of concessions to the prejudices or the preferences of the members. Whoever reads these privately-printed lectures can take them to represent Anthroposophy in the fullest sense. Thus it was possible without hesitation—when the complaints in this direction became too persistent—to depart from the custom of circulating this material only among members. But it must be borne in mind that faulty passages occur in these lecture-reports not revised by myself.

The right to judge such private material can of course, be conceded only to someone who has the pre-requisite basis for such judgment. And in respect of most of this material it would mean *at least* knowledge of man and of the cosmos insofar as these have been presented in the light of Anthroposophy, and also knowledge of what exists as "anthroposophical history" in what has been imparted from the spiritual world.'

SPEECH EURYTHMY COURSE

REPORT IN THE "NEWS-SHEET"
(NACHRICHTENBLATT)

20th July 1924

From June 24th—July 12th a course of lectures on speech eurythmy was held at the Goetheanum. It had as content a further presentation of much which had already been given in this domain and at the same time a deepening and widening of what was already known. The eurythmy artists, who both at the Goetheanum and going out from there to many places, are practicing eurythmy as an art, the eurythmy teachers, the teaching staff of the Stuttgart eurythmy school founded and directed by Marie Steiner, the eurythmy teachers of the Waldorf School and the Fortbildungsschule at the Goetheanum, the curative eurythmists, and a number of personalities who through their profession as artists or scientists in other spheres are interested in eurythmy, attended the course.

Eurythmy makes it possible to bring the artistic as such, in its essence and its sources, to visible beholding. This was specially borne in mind during the presentation of this course. He only can work as eurythmy artist who creatively unfolds a sense for art from an inner call, an inner enthusiasm.

In order to bring to manifestation the possibilities of form and movement inherent in the human organisation it is necessary that the soul be completely enfilled with art. This universal character of eurythmy underlay all that was presented.

Whoever wishes to do eurythmy must have penetrated into the being of speech-formation. He must, before all, have approached the mysteries of sound-creation. In every sound an expression for a soul experience is given; in the vowel-sounds for a thinking, feeling, willing self-revelation of the soul, in the consonant sounds for the way in which the soul represents an outer thing or a process. This

9

expression of language remains for the most part quite subconscious in the case of ordinary speech; the eurythmist must learn to know it quite exactly, for he has to transform what becomes audible in speech into gestures which are quiescent or in movement. In this course, therefore, the inner structure of language was revealed. The sound-significance of the word, which everywhere underlies the meaning-significance, was made visible. By the eurythmy gestures themselves, some aspects of the inner laws of language—little recognised at the present time, when speaking is the expression of a strongly abstract attitude of soul—can be visibly manifested. That is what happened in this course. Thereby, it may be hoped, it will also have given to eurythmy teachers the guiding lines necessary for them.

The eurythmist must devote himself to the gesture down to its smallest detail, so that his performance really becomes the self-understood expression of the life of soul. He can only give form to the gesture in its fullness when the smallest detail comes first to consciousness, that it may later become the habitual expression of the soul-being.

A study was made of how the gesture as such reveals soul-experience and spirit-content, and also of how this revelation relates itself to the soul-expression which is manifested audibly in the language of sound. From eurythmy one can learn to value the technique of art; but from eurythmy one can indeed also become deeply imbued with the way in which the technical must put aside everything external and be completely taken hold of by the soul, if the truly artistic is to come to life. People who are active in any sphere of art often speak of how the soul must work *behind* the technique; the truth is that it is *in* the technique that the soul must work.

A special value was laid in these lectures upon showing that in the truly formed gestures the aesthetically sensitive human being perceives the soul-element directly in a quite unequivocal way. Examples were shown which demonstrated how a content in the soul-configuration can be made obvious in a certain gesture-formation.

10

It was also shown how the whole structure of language, which reveals itself in grammar, syntax, rhythm, in poetical figures of speech, in rhyme and verse-formation, also finds its corresponding realisation in eurythmy.

The audience attending this course was not only to be led into the knowledge of eurythmy but they should be brought to the experience of how all art must be sustained by love and enthusiasm. The eurythmist cannot separate himself from his artistic creation and objectively put it forward for aesthetic enjoyment as can the painter or sculptor, but he remains personally within his performance; one *sees* from him himself whether or no art lives within him as a divine world-content. In the immediate artistic present, art in its visible essence must be made manifest by the actual human being of the eurythmist. This demands a particularly inward and intimate relationship to art. To help the partakers towards *this* understanding was the aim of this course. It wished to show how, when beholding the gestures, feeling, inner perception is enkindled in the soul, and how this inner perception then leads to the experience of the visible word. Much which can only be partially expressed in the audible word can be completely revealed through the movements of eurythmy. The audible word in recitation and declamation, in conjunction with the visible word, produces a total expression which can result in the most intensive artistic unity.

SYNOPSIS OF LECTURES

I. EURYTHMY AS VISIBLE SPEECH

It is necessary for the eurythmist to be able to enter into eurythmy with his whole personality, with his whole being, so that this art may become an expression of life itself. When we wish to penetrate into the nature of eurythmy we have to do with a penetration into the being of man. Eurythmy must be a creation out of the spirit and must make use of human movement as its means of expression. Speech itself is not the imitation of anything, and eurythmy also must represent an original creation. ' In the beginning was the Word.' Primeval humanity conceived ' the Word ' as comprising in itself the entire human being as etheric creation. This human etheric body is in continual movement, ever taking on new forms; these forms are only to be captured when the whole content of speech is uttered aloud and thus given shape. These sound-forms which issue from the larynx are inherent in the formation of the larynx and its neighbouring organs. When we utter a word we produce a definite form in the air. If we were able to utter the alphabet from *a* to *z*, in such a way that the whole could take shape in the air, we should have the form of the human etheric body. This etheric body contains within it the forces of growth, of nourishment and of memory; all this is imparted to the air when we speak. In this way words arise. The etheric man is the word which comprises the whole alphabet. That which comes into being through speech is the birth of the etheric man. In the sound of each individual word some part of the human being is contained. Everything in the world is a part of us. Nothing exists which may not find expression through the human being. In the creative larynx we have the etheric man as an air form in a state of

12

becoming. Spoken words are always a partial birth of the etheric man. When we speak we have to do with an etheric creation of the human being. In speech we are faced with a creative activity welling up from the depths of universal life. Speech is bound up with the origin of the human being. Human knowledge begins with wonder, with *a;* in *b* we have the protecting sheath; every sound tells us something about man; when we arrive at the sound *z* we have a synthesis of human wisdom. Nearly the whole life of the soul, in its aspect of feeling, is expressed in *i, o, a.* These possibilities of movement when held fast give us the physical form of man. This perfected form arose out of movement, out of primeval forms which continually came into being and again dissolved. Movement does not arise out of that which is at rest; the form at rest arises out of movement. The human form is the result of a divine eurythmy. Every art may be traced back to a divine source; but because eurythmy makes use of the human being as its instrument it enables us to see most deeply into the connection between the human being and the universe.

2. THE CHARACTER OF THE INDIVIDUAL SOUNDS

Consonants: an imitation of external happenings; vowels: an inner experience; *h*: midway between the consonants and the vowels in its relation to the breath; for the breath is partially an inward experience and in part streams outwards. Primeval language. The nature of the individual sounds.

3. THE GESTURES; HOW THEY ARE FORMED AND EXPERIENCED

The mood and feeling contained in the sounds: *s, z, a, e, u, ei, b, c, d, f, l, m, n, z.* An explanation of the way in which, by means of eurythmy, the experiences underlying the gestures may be carried over into their actual form.

13

4. THE INDIVIDUAL SOUNDS AND THEIR COMBINATION INTO WORDS

The inner nature of the sounds was revealed in the ancient Mysteries. The different characteristics of language; for instance the German language is a sculptor, the Magyar language a hunter.—Eurythmy is a language which may be understood if approached without prejudice. The sounds are the essential basis of eurythmy; special attention must be paid to the transition from one sound to another. By means of eurythmy it is possible to enter into the living spirit of language and to experience the essential nature of words.—In the Russian language one is always following on the tracks of the word; in the French language the movement is always in advance of the word. One may pass over from the nature of individual words to the inner logic contained in language. In this logic the character of the different peoples is brought to expression.

5. THE MOOD AND FEELING OF A POEM

Transition from the actual sounds to the logical or emotional content of speech. Emphasis. The question mark, exclamation mark, merriment, cleverness, knowledge, self-assertion, frenzy, insatiability, inwardness, charm, the bringing of tidings, sadness, despair. By means of these gestures different moods of soul may be brought to plastic-eurythmic expression.

6. DIFFERENT ASPECTS OF THE SOUL LIFE. THE INNER NATURE OF COLOUR

Description of gestures which are drawn out of the whole human organization and which express some underlying mood. Devotion, solemnity. The three categories of the

14

life of the soul: Thinking, Feeling, Willing. The more intimate nature of a poem is expressed by means of the treatment of language. The use of the *e*-sound by poets tending more towards thought, the epic; the use of the sounds *a, e, u,* when the tendency is towards feeling; the use of many consonants when will is predominant. Straight and curved lines.—Significance of sound when choosing colour of dress and veil. It is only possible to enter truly into the nature of a sound when the corresponding colours are experienced. Colour is the life of the soul transfixed in the outer world. Every human being has a fundamental colour.

7. THE PLASTIC FORMATION OF SPEECH

The structure of language as such and the character of the separate sounds must be brought to visible form in eurythmy. The ' air-gestures ' which may be said to be present in language are imitated and made externally visible. The consonant sounds are adapted to a more plastic interpretation. The character of the breath sounds is a yielding to the outer world. In the consonants of force man confronts the outer world as master; these sounds are an assertion of the inner life. Movement as such is expressed in the vibrating and wave-like sounds. The diphthongs: it is here that one best learns to observe the transition from one sound to another; the first sound is arrested when half completed and led over into the last half of the movement for the second sound. We weld the component parts together when we do not allow either to be fully formed. The diphthong has no sharply defined outlines; a feeling of plurality is given when the diphthong is fundamental to the structure of the word. When an impression is indefinite the diphthong makes its appearance. It is possible for eurythmy to bring to expression the inner character of sound. *I, e, u,* radiate a Dionysian fire. *A, o,* have a quiet power of attraction, an Apollonian form-giving element.

15

8. THE WORD AS DEFINITION AND THE WORD IN ITS CONTEXT

In the realm of sound we may differentiate between that which descends more into the physical and that which is borne upwards by the word into the spiritual world. When a vowel sound becomes a diphthong, thus losing its sharply defined outline, we have an ascent into the spiritual. The diphthongs reveal something of a more essentially spiritual nature than do the vowel sounds of which they are composed. That element of language which radiates up towards the spiritual does not lie in the sharply emphasized sound, but in the transition from one sound to the other. The dual nature of words: on the one side external imitation; on the other side the depicting of something in its connection with the entire world order, the relationship of some thing or process to a common whole. Personal pronouns and their forms.

9. PLASTIC SPEECH

Walking as the expression of an impulse of will. Three phases: the lifting, carrying and placing of the foot. When *lifting* the foot we have to do with a will impulse as such; when *carrying* the foot with the thought which comes to expression in this will-impulse; and when *placing* the foot with the deed, with the fulfilment of the will-impulse. Rhythmic walking; poetic and prose language. The true nature of speech lies midway between thought and feeling. Man at an earlier stage of evolution *heard* inwardly when experiencing feeling; he had an inner experience of words. His was no abstract thought but an inner resounding of words. There was no self-contained life of feeling such as we have to-day; the primitive soul life was closely bound up with the inner configuration of words and tones. At one time the development of speech, thought and feeling was deeply connected with an inner recitation. Later this differentiated itself into language retaining its artistic nature, and into a musical, wordless resounding of tones. Then thought

16

as a third element also took on independent existence. Because the prose element of abstract thought is closely bound up with materialism, there is to-day little feeling for an artistic treatment of language.

The eurythmist must be able to acquire this. In the first place there must be a feeling for the Iambic and Trochaic rhythms, for these impart a special character to walking: the Iambic measure expresses the will character, the Trochaic measure the realization of thought. In the Anapest we have a more intimate aspect of language, one more bound up with the feeling life; it is a spiritualization of language. When the Trochaic is developed further we get the Dactyl measure, —an announcement, a statement, an assertion, made visible in space and time. By means of these movements in space one can enter into the poetic element in language more easily than in the case of recitation or declamation. In the artistic formation of speech one must endeavour to cultivate imagination and fantasy, for the inner formation of language depends upon the possibility of making pictures. A sound as such is always the picture of what it describes; anyone feeling this will develop in himself a feeling for the use of the pictorial in poetic language. Metaphor. Synecdoche. Walking backwards: an ascent towards that which is more comprehensive; walking forwards: the entering into that which is less comprehensive. Walking sideways: a conversation, for conversation has a metaphor formation, inasmuch as it has to do with the relationship between two things.

10. MOVEMENTS ARISING OUT OF THE BEING OF MAN

Up to this point the character of the eurythmy gestures has arisen out of the sounds of speech; we will now take our start from the being of man and develop other possibilities of movement and gesture. Twelve gestures which in their totality represent the whole being of man. They comprise all the qualities which together make up the human being

17

and weld them into one whole in the Zodiac. In these postures and gestures the human faculties are brought to expression. From these static postures we pass over to movements representing the possibilities of inner activity, movements which have their origin in the planets. In their sevenfold nature we have synthesized the animal element in man. The nineteen possibilities of sound: the consonants have their source in the Zodiac; the vowels in the dance of the planets. A cosmic activity may be brought to expression by means of human gesture and movement. The word of the heavens is really the being of man. By means of an imitation of the dance of the stars, discovered through spiritual knowledge, we have the possibility of renewing in eurythmy the temple dancing of the ancient Mysteries.

11. HOW ONE MAY ENTER INTO THE NATURE OF GESTURE AND FORM

Looking at speech from a spiritual aspect we find that what is of the most importance lies between the sounds. The spirit is manifested at the point of transition from one sound to another. Hence the movements must always be carried out with a deep feeling and inwardness. The essential spirituality underlying certain postures and movements must be brought out in the way in which the sounds are formed. Exercises based on the moving circles of the Zodiac and Planets and their corresponding spiritual gestures. Such exercises bring the eurythmic movements and postures right down in to the organism.

12. THE OUTPOURING OF THE HUMAN SOUL INTO FORM AND MOVEMENT: THE CURATIVE EFFECT OF THIS UPON THE MORAL AND PSYCHIC LIFE AND ITS REACTION UPON THE WHOLE BEING OF MAN

In the numbers Twelve and Seven we have brought certain moral impulses before our souls and these find expression in gestures which are either static or mobile. That which streams out in this way works back on to the human being;

this is the basis of the curative effect of eurythmy. The effect of such curative methods upon the moral and psychic life will be especially beneficial when certain eurythmic truths are brought to the human being in childhood. With this in view we choose exercises in which form and content have been developed out of certain conditions of soul, exercises which are then able to react curatively. ' I and Thou' exercise: excellent for educational purposes. Peace Dance, Energy Dance. The spiral forms.

13. MOODS OF SOUL WHICH ARISE OUT OF THE GESTURES FOR THE SOUNDS

Special character of certain eurythmic exercises: Hallelujah, Evoe. Irony as revealed by the gesture itself. Eurythmy forms may be made the basis of poetic structure. In certain Mystery Centres poetry arose out of gesture and form. The movements and forms of eurythmy preceded the shaping of a poem. True poetry always has eurythmy within it; it is as though the poet first carried out the corresponding movements and gestures in his etheric body. Herein we find the intimate connection between eurythmy and language. The use of accelerated and retarded tempo.

14. THE STRUCTURE OF WORDS. THE INNER STRUCTURE OF VERSE.

In order to make the structure of language intelligible it is necessary to divide words into categories according to the train of thought. This also must be taken into account in eurythmy. We must differentiate between nouns, adjectives, verbs, prepositions, etc., with their individual characteristics. Example of a form corresponding to a four-lined verse. The eurythmist can acquire a fine and delicate understanding for the secrets of the human organization by means of the meditation given in this lecture.

15. IN EURYTHMY THE BODY MUST BECOME SOUL

An inner strengthening by means of the g-sound. In the w-sound (English v) there lies the feeling of a moving shelter; this is the sound most naturally used in alliteration.—Difference between standing and walking: one imitates something when standing still; when walking one desires actually to *be* something. Poetry for the most part expresses what is living, the actual *being* of a thing, not what it signifies.—Connection of the human body with the whole cosmos; the feet are suited to the earth; hands and arms express the soul nature. It is the soul life especially which is brought to expression in eurythmy; this is why the most significant part of eurythmy is the movement of the arms and hands; the head expresses the spirit and, according to its organization, can be made use of in many ways.—The twelve movements connected with the Zodiac and the seven movements connected with the moving circle of the Planets may be variously applied. They may be used, for instance, to show the rhyme.—Harmonizing exercises: ' Ich denke die Rede.'— The necessity of carefully analysing what is to be expressed in eurythmy; it is of more importance to study the sound-content than the sense-content. The eurythmist must first experience the formation and structure of the sounds of a poem and only later bring it to eurythmic expression. Movement, Feeling, Character. The soul must learn, as far as eurythmy is concerned, actually to live in the body. In eurythmy the whole body must become soul.

LECTURE 1

Dornach, 24th June 1924

These lectures dealing with the nature of eurythmy are given in response to a request from Frau Dr. Steiner, who believes it to be necessary, in order to lay the foundation of an exact eurythmic tradition, to recapitulate in the first place all that has been given in the domain of speech-eurythmy at different times to different people. To this repetition fresh material will be added in order to widen the field of eurythmic expression. Such material will, however, not be set apart in separate chapters, but will be given in connection with each individual point as this comes under discussion.

I shall endeavour to deal with eurythmy from its various aspects; not only from the artistic side which naturally calls for our first consideration here, but also from the point of view of education and healing.

The first lecture will be in the nature of an introduction and this will be followed by a lecture dealing with the first elements of speech-eurythmy. In every branch of eurythmic activity it is necessary above all that the personality, the whole human being of the eurythmist should be brought into play, so that eurythmy may become an expression of life itself. This cannot be achieved unless one enters into the spirit of eurythmy, feeling it actually as visible speech. As in the case of all artistic appreciation, it is quite possible for anyone to enjoy eurythmy as a spectator, without having acquired any knowledge of its essential basis, just as it is quite unnecessary to have studied harmony or counterpoint to be able to appreciate music. For it is an accepted fact of human evolution that the healthily developed human being carries within him a natural appreciation and understanding of art.

21

Art must work through its own inherent power. Art must explain itself. Those, however, who are studying eurythmy, whose duty it is in some way or another to bring eurythmy before the world, must penetrate into the actual essence and nature of eurythmy in just the same way as, let us say, the musician, the painter or the sculptor must enter into the nature of his own particular art. If we wish to enter into the true nature of eurythmy we must perforce enter into the true nature of the human being. For eurythmy, to a far greater extent than any other art, makes use of what lies in the nature of man himself. Take for example various other arts, arts which need instruments or tools for their expression. You find no instrument or tool so nearly akin to the human being as the instrument made use of by the eurythmist. The art of mime and the art of dancing do indeed to some extent make use of the human being as a means of artistic expression. With the art of mime, however, that which is expressed through the mime itself is merely subordinate to the performance as a whole, for such a performance does not depend entirely upon the artistic, plastic use of the human being. In such a case this same human being is made use of in order to imitate something or other which is already represented in man here upon the earth.

Further, in the case of the art of mime, we find as a rule that the gestures are used mainly to emphasize and render clearer something which is made use of by man in everyday life; that is to say, mime emphasizes speech. In order to bring a more intimate note into speech, gesture is added. Thus we are here concerned with something which merely adds in some small measure to the scope of that which is already present in man on the physical plane.

In the art of dancing—if we may use the word ' art ' in such a connection when dancing rises to the level of art—we have to do with an outpouring of the emotions, of the will, into movements of the human body, whereby are only further developed those possibilities of movement inherent in the human being and already present elsewhere on the physical plane. In eurythmy we have to do with

22

something which can nowhere be found in the human being in ordinary physical life, but which must be through and through a creation out of the spiritual worlds. We have to do with something which makes use of the human being, which makes use of the human form and its movement as a means of expression.

Now the question arises:—What *is* really expressed in eurythmy?—This you will only understand when you begin to realize that eurythmy is actually a visible speech. With regard to speech itself the following must be said. When we give form to speech by means of mime, the ordinary speech itself provides us with a picture, with an image; when, however, we give form to speech *itself*, to sound as such, we find that the latter contains within it no such image. Speech arises as a separate, independent product from out of the human being himself. Nowhere in Nature do we find that which reveals itself in speech, that which comes into being through speech.

For this reason eurythmy must, in its very nature, be something which represents a primeval creation. Speech—let us take this as our starting point—speech appears as a production of the human larynx and of those organs of speech which are more or less connected with it. What is the nature of the larynx? This question must eventually be brought forward, for I have often shown how in eurythmy the whole human being must become a sort of larynx. We must therefore put to ourselves the question: Of what significance is the larynx? Now if you look upon speech merely as a production of the larynx, you will gain no conception of what is really proceeding from it, of what is being fashioned within it, Here it would perhaps be well to remind ourselves of a remarkable tradition which to-day is little understood, and of which you find some indication when you take the beginning of St. John's Gospel: ' In the Beginning was the Word, and the Word was with God, and a God was the Word .' The Word.—Of course that which we to-day imagine to be the Word is something which gives not the slightest sense to the opening sentences of this Gospel. Nevertheless they are continually quoted. People believe they can make something out of them. They do not, however, succeed. For it is an undeniable fact that the conception of a word as held by the man of to-day is often truly expressed by his saying something of this kind:—What is a name but mere sound and smoke, mist and vapour?—In a certain sense he values the word itself little in comparison with its underlying concept. He feels a certain superiority in thus being able to value the word little in comparison with the thought. When, therefore, one puts oneself in the position of the man of to-day, and considers his conception of a word, the beginning of St. John's Gospel has indeed no meaning. For consider: the Word?— we have so many words, which word? It can only be a definite, concrete word. And what is the nature of this Word? That is the question.

Now behind this tradition which is indicated in the beginning of this Gospel lies the fact that man once had an instinctive knowledge of the true nature of the Word. To-day, however, this knowledge has been lost. To primeval human understanding the idea, the conception, ' the Word ' comprised *the whole human being as an etheric creation.*

All of you, as Anthroposophists, know what we mean by the etheric man. We have the physical man and we have the etheric man. Physical man, as he is described to-day by modern physiology and anatomy, consists, both outwardly and inwardly, of certain forms which can be drawn. Here, however, one naturally does not take into consideration the fact that what one draws is only the very smallest part of the physical human being, for the physical body is at the same time fluidic; it consists also of air and warmth. These constituents are naturally not included when one is speaking of the human being in physiology and anatomy. Nevertheless it is possible to gain some idea of the nature of the physical body of man.

We have, however, the second member of the human being, —the etheric body. If we were to attempt to draw the etheric body something extraordinarily complicated would come to expression. For the etheric body can just as little be represented as something static as can lightning. It is impossible to paint lightning; for lightning is in continual movement, lightning is in continual flow. In portraying lightning one must attempt to show it in continual flow and movement. And the same holds good with the etheric body. The etheric body is in continual motion, in continual activity.

Now these movements, these gestures which are continually in movement,—of which the etheric body does not indeed consist, but out of which it continually arises and again passes away,—do we find them anywhere in the world of man, do we come up against them anywhere? Yes, we do. This was no secret to a primeval and intuitive knowledge. We have these movements,—and here, my dear friends, I must ask you to take what I am saying quite literally,—we have these movements in the sound formations which embody the content of speech.

Now review mentally all the sounds of speech to which your larynx gives form and utterance, inasmuch as this formative principle is applied to the entire range of articulate speech. Bear in mind all the component elements which issue from the larynx for the purpose of speech. You must realise that all these elements, proceeding as they do from the larynx, really form the component parts of that which is brought to outer expression in speech. You must realise that these sound-formations consist of definite movements, the origin of which lies in the structure and form of the larynx and its neighbouring organs. They proceed from the larynx.

But these movements do not of course appear simultaneously. We cannot utter all the sounds which make up the content of speech at the same moment. How then could we utter all that makes up the content of speech? We could do so,—paradoxical as this may sound it is nevertheless a fact,—we could do so if for once we were to utter one after the other all the possible sounds from *a*, *b*, *c*, down to *z*. Try to imagine this. Imagine that someone were to say the alphabet aloud, beginning with *a*, *b* and continuing as far as *z*, with only the necessary pauses for breathing. Every spoken sound describes a certain form in the air, which one does not see but the existence of which must be pre-supposed. It is possible, indeed, to think of these forms being retained, fixed by scientific means, without actually making a physical drawing of them.

When we utter any particular word aloud,—' tree ' for example, or ' sun ',—we produce a quite definite air-form.

If we were to say the whole alphabet aloud from a to z, we should produce a very complicated air-form. Let us put this question to ourselves:—What really would be the result if someone were actually to do this? It would have to take place within a certain time,—as you will learn in the course of these lectures. It would have to take place within a certain time, so that, on reaching z, the first sound would not have completely disintegrated, that is to say the a-sound must still retain its plastic form when we have reached the sound z. If it were actually possible in this creation of air-forms to pass from a to z in such a way that the a-sound remained when the z-sound were reached, thus creating in the air an image of the whole alphabet, what would be the result? What sort of form should we have made? We should have created the form of the human etheric body. In this way we should have reproduced the human etheric body. If you were to repeat the alphabet aloud from a to z —(one would have to do this in exactly the right way; the alphabetical order of sounds in general use to-day is no longer quite correct—but I am speaking now of the under-lying principle)—the human etheric body would stand before you.

What then would really have taken place? The human etheric body is always present. Every man bears it within himself. What do you do therefore when you speak, when you say the alphabet aloud? You sink so to speak, into the form of your own etheric body. What happens then, when we utter a single word, which of course does not consist of all the sounds? Let us picture to ourselves the human being as he stands before us. He consists of physical body, etheric body, astral body and ego. He speaks some

26

word. He sinks his consciousness into his etheric body. He forms some part of the etheric body in the air as an image, in much the same way as you, standing before a physical body, might for instance copy the form of a hand, so that the form of the hand were made visible in the air. Now the etheric body does not consist of the same forms as those which make up the physical body, but in this case it is the forms of the etheric body which are impressed into the air. When we learn to understand this rightly, my dear friends, we gain an insight into the most wonderful metamorphosis of the human form, an insight into the evolution of man. For what is this etheric body? It is the vehicle of the forces of growth; it contains within it all those forces bound up with the processes of nourishment, and also those forces connected with the power of memory. All this is imparted to the airy formations when we speak.

The inner being of man, in so far as this is expressed in the etheric body, is impressed into the air when we speak. When we put sounds together, words arise. When we put together the whole alphabet from beginning to end, there arises a very complicated word. This word contains every possibility of word-formation. It also contains at the same time the human being in his etheric nature. Before man appeared on the earth as a physical being he already existed as an etheric being. For the etheric man underlies the physical man. How then may the etheric man be described? The etheric man is the Word which contains within it the entire alphabet.

Thus when we are able to speak of the formation of this primeval Word, which existed from the beginning before physical man came into being, we find that that which arises in connection with speech may indeed be called a birth,—a birth of the whole etheric man when the alphabet is spoken aloud. Otherwise, in the single words, it is a partial birth, a birth of fragments, of parts of the human being. In every single word as it is uttered there lies something of the being of man. Let us take the word 'tree' for instance,—what does it mean when we say the word 'tree'?

When we say the word ' tree ' it means that we describe the tree in some such way as this. We say: That which stands there in the outer world, to which we give the name ' tree ' is a part of ourselves, a part of our own etheric being. Everything in the world is a part of ourselves; nothing exists which cannot be expressed through the being of man. Just as the human being when he gives utterance to the whole alphabet really gives utterance to *himself*, and consequently to the whole universe, so, when uttering single words, which represent fragments of the Collective Word, of the alphabet, he gives expression to something which is a part of the universe. The entire universe would be expressed if the whole alphabet were uttered from beginning to end. Parts of the universe are expressed in the single words.

There is one thing, however, about which we must be quite clear when we think over all that lies behind sound as such. Behind sound as such there lies everything that is comprised in the inner being of man. The activity manifested by the etheric body is representative of inner experiences of the soul in the nature of feeling. We must now find our way to these feelings themselves which are experienced in the human soul.

Let us take the sound *a* as a beginning.* To-day one learns to utter the sound *a* when one is in that unconscious dreamy condition in which one lives as a very small child. This experience is later buried when the child suffers harm at school as a result of receiving wrong teaching in sound and language. When one learns to speak as a child there

* Owing to the fact that a number of German examples and quotations have had to be retained in the translation of these lectures, the German pronunciation of the vowel sounds has been consistently used throughout.

German *a*, English *ah* (as in father)
	e,	„	*a* („ „ say)
	i,	„	*ee* („ „ feet)
	ei,	„	*i*, („ „ light)
	au,	„	*ow* („ „ how)
	eu,	„	*oi* („ „ joy)

28

is really present something of the great mystery of speech. It remains, however, in a state of dreamy unconsciousness.

When we utter the sound *a* we feel, if our instinct is at all healthy, that this sound really proceeds from our inmost being when we are in a state of *wonder* and *amazement*.

Now this wonder is of course again only a part of the human being. Man is no abstraction. At every *waking* moment of his life he is something or other. One can of course allow oneself to become sluggish or stupefied, in which case one cannot be said to be anything very definite. But the human being must always be *something*, even when he reduces himself to a state of torpor; at every minute of the day he must be something or other. Now he is filled with wonder, now with fear, or again, let us say, with aggressive activity. The human being is no abstraction; every second he must be something definite. Thus there are times when man is a being of wonder, a being filled with amazement. The processes at work in the etheric body when man experiences wonder are imprinted into the air with the help of the larynx when he utters the sound *a*. When man utters the sound *a* he sends forth out of himself a part of his own being, namely the quality of wonder. This he imprints into the air.

We know that when a physical man appears upon the earth, he appears,—if he is born in accordance with the ordinary possibilities of development,—as a complete human being. This complete human being comes forth from the womb of the mother. He is born as physical man with a physical form. If all the sounds of the alphabet were uttered from *a* to *z* there would arise an etheric man, only this etheric man would be imprinted into the air, born from out of the human larynx and its neighbouring organs.

In the same way, when the child is brought into the world, when the child first sees the light, we must say: From out of the womb and its neighbouring organs there has arisen a physical man.

But the larynx differs from the womb of the mother in that it is in a continual state of creation. So that in single words

29

fragments of the human being arise; and indeed, if one were to bring together all the words of a language (—which even in the case of a poet of such rich vocabulary as Shakespeare never actually occurs—) the entire etheric man as an air-form would be produced by means of the creative larynx, but it would be a succession of births, a continuous becoming. It would be a birth continually taking place during the process of speech. Speech is always the bringing to birth of parts of the etheric man.

Again the physical larynx is only the external sheath of that most wonderful organ which is present in the etheric body, and which is, as it were, the womb of the Word. And here again we are confronted with a wonderful metamorphosis. Everything which is present in the human being is a metamorphosis of certain fundamental forms. The etheric larynx and its sheath, the physical larynx, are a metamorphosis of the uterus. In speech we have to do with the creation of man, with the creation of man as an etheric being.

This mystery of speech, my dear friends, is indicated by the connection which we find between the vocal and sexual functions, a connection clearly illustrated in the breaking of the male voice.

We have therefore to do with a creative activity which, welling up from the depths of cosmic life, flows outwards through the medium of speech. We see revealed in a fluctuating, ever-changing form that which otherwise withdraws itself into the mysterious depths of the human organization at the moment of physical birth. Thus we gain something which is essential for us in our artistic creative activity. We gain respect, reverence, for that creative element into which we, as artists, are placed. Theoretical discussion is useless in the realm of art. We cannot do with it; it merely leads us into abstraction. In art we need something which places us with our whole human being into the cosmic being. And how could we penetrate more deeply into the cosmic being than by becoming conscious of the relation existing between speech and the genesis of man. Every time that a man speaks he produces out of himself some part of that which existed in primeval times, when the human being was created out of cosmic depths, out of the etheric forces, and received form as a being of air before he acquired fluidic form, and, later still, his solid physical form. Every time we speak we transpose ourselves into the cosmic evolution of man as it was in primeval ages.

Let us take an example. Let us go back once more to the sound *a*, this sound which calls up within us the human being in a state of wonder. We must realize that every time the sound *a* appears in language there lies behind it the element of wonder. Let us take the word *Wasser* (water), or the word *Pfahl* (post), any word you like in which the sound *a* occurs. In every instance, when you lay stress on the sound *a* in speech, there lies in the background a feeling of wonder; the human being filled with wonder is brought to expression in this way by means of speech. There was a time when this was known. It was, for example, known to the Hebraic people. For what really lay behind the *a*, the Aleph, in the Hebrew language? What was the Aleph? It was wonder as manifested in the human being.

Now I should like to remind you of something which could lead you to an understanding of all that is really indicated by the sound *a*, all that the sound *a* really signifies. In ancient Greece there was a saying: Philosophy begins with wonder. Philosophy, the love of wisdom, the love of knowledge, begins with wonder.—Had one spoken absolutely organically, really in accordance with primeval understanding, with primeval instinctive—clairvoyant understanding, one might equally well have said:—Philosophy begins with *a*.—To a primeval humanity this would have meant exactly the same thing.— Philosophy, love of wisdom begins with *a*.

But what is it that one is really investigating when one studies philosophy? When all is said and done one is really investigating man. Philosophy strives after self-knowledge, and this self-observation begins with the sound *a*. It is, however, at the same time a most profound mystery, for it requires great effort, great activity, to attain to such knowledge of the human being. When man approaches his own being and sees how it is formed out of body, soul and spirit, when he looks upon his own being in its entirety, then he is confronted by something before which he may say *a* with the deepest wonder. For this reason *a* corresponds to man in a state of wonder, to man filled with wonder at his own true being, that is to say, man looked at from the highest, most ideal aspect.

The realization that man, as he stands before us as a physical being, is but a part of the complete human being, and that we only have the real man before us when we perceive the full measure of the divinity within him,—this realization, this wonder called up in us by a contemplation of our own being, was called by a primeval humanity: *A*. *A* corresponds to man in his highest perfection. Thus *A* is man, and in the sound *a* we are expressing something which is felt in the depths of the human soul. Let us pass over from *a* to *b*, in order to give at least some indication of that which might lead to an understanding of this primeval word which is made up of the entire alphabet. Let us pass over to *b*. In *b* we have a so-called consonant; in *a* we have to do with a vowel sound. You will feel, if you pronounce a vowel-sound, that you are giving expression to something coming from the inmost depths of your own being. Every vowel, as we have already seen in the case of the vowel *a*, is bound up with an experience of the soul. In every case where the sound *a* makes its appearance, we have the feeling of wonder. In every case where an *e* makes its appearance we have an experience which can be expressed somewhat as follows:— *I become aware that something has been done to me.*

Just think for a moment what creatures of abstraction we have become, how withered and lifeless our nature. Just as an apple or a plum may shrivel up, so have we become shrivelled up as regards our experience of language. Let us consider how, in speaking, when we pronounce the sound *a* and proceed from this sound to the sound *e* (which constantly happens) we have no idea that we are passing over from the feeling of wonder to the feeling: I become aware that something has been done to me.—Let us now enter into the feeling of the *i*-sound. With *i* we have, as it were, the feeling that we have been curious about something and that our curiosity has been satisfied. A wonderful and far from simple experience lies at the back of every vowel-sound. When we allow the five vowel-sounds to work upon us we receive the impression of man in his primeval strength and vigour. Man is, as it were, born again in his true dignity when he allows these five sounds consciously to work upon him, that is to say when he allows these sounds to proceed out of his inmost being in full consciousness. Therefore it is true to say:—We have become quite shrivelled up and think only of the meaning of a word, utterly disregarding the experience behind it. We think only of the meaning. The word ' water ' for instance means some particular thing and so on. We have become utterly shrivelled up.

The consonants are quite different in their nature from the vowels. With the consonants we do not feel that the sounds arise from our inmost experience, but we feel that they are images of that which is outside our own being.

Let us suppose that I am filled with wonder, that I say *a*. I cannot make an outer image of the sound *a*, I must give utterance to it. If, however, I would give expression to something which is round in its form, like this table, for example, what must I do if I do not wish to express it in words? I must imitate it, I must copy its form, (corresponding gesture). If I would describe a nose without speaking, without actually saying the word ' nose ' but still wishing to make myself understood, I can, as it were, copy its form, (corresponding gesture). And it is just the same in the forming of the consonants. In the consonants we have an imitation of that which exists in the external world. They are always an imitation of external forms. But we express these forms by constructing them in the air, producing them by means of the larynx and its neighbouring organs, the palate, for example. With the help of these organs we create a form which imitates, copies something which exists outside ourselves. This is even carried into the actual form of the letters, but of this we shall speak later.

33

When we form a *b* (it is, by the way, impossible to pronounce this sound without the addition of some vowel) when we form a *b* it is the imitation of something in the external world. If we were able to hold fast the air-form which is created by *b* (we must, of course, speak the sound aloud) we should have something in the nature of a *shelter*. A protecting, sheltering form would be produced. Something would be produced which might be likened to a hut or a house. *B* is an imitation of a house. Thus when we begin with *a*, *b*, we have, as it were, the human being in his perfection, and the human being in his house: *a*, *b*.

And so, if we were to go through the whole alphabet, we should, in the consecutive sounds, unfold the mystery of man. We should express the human being as he lives in the cosmos, the human being in his house, his physical sheath. If we were to pass from *a*, *b*, to *c*, *d*, and so on, every sound would tell us something about the human being. And on reaching *z* we should have pictured in sound the whole of human wisdom, for this is contained in the etheric body of man.

We see from this that something of the very greatest significance takes place in speech. In speech the human being himself is fashioned. And one can indeed give a fairly complete picture of the soul life of man when one brings to expression his most fundamental feelings. *I*, *O*, *A*. These sounds represent practically the whole content of the human soul in its aspect of feeling: *I*, *O*, *A*.

Let us for a moment consider all that proceeds from the human being when he speaks. Let us suppose that somebody repeats the alphabet; when this is done the entire etheric body of man comes into being, proceeding from the larynx, as from the womb. The etheric body is brought into being. When we look at the physical body of man we know that it has come forth from the organism of the mother, it has come forth from a metamorphosis of the larynx, that is to say, from the mother's womb.

But now let us picture to ourselves, the complete human being as he comes into the world with all his different attributes; for that which is brought forth from the organism of the mother cannot remain unchanged. If the human being were to remain unchanged through his whole life, he could not be said to be a man in the true sense of the word; one thing must be continually added to another. The human being at the age of thirty-five, let us say, has gained more from the universal, cosmic being than was his as a child. We may picture the whole human being in some such way as this. Just as speech proceeds from out of the larynx, the child from out of the womb, so the fully developed human being at about the age of thirty-five is born, as it were, from out of the cosmos in the same way in which the words which we speak are spoken out of us. Thus we have the form of man, the complete human form, as a spoken word.

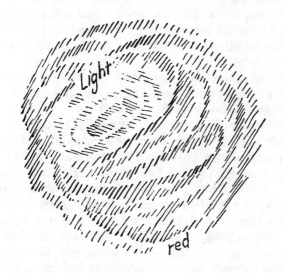

The human form stands before us,—that most wonderful of earthly forms,—the human form stands before us and we ask the divine spiritual powers which have existed from the beginning: How then did you create man in a similar way as the spoken word is created when we speak? How did you

35

create man? What really took place when you created man?—And if we were to receive an answer to our question from out of universal space, it would be some such answer as this: All around us there is movement, form, constantly changing and of infinite variety: such a form (*a* was here shown in eurythmy), such a form (*e* was shown), such a form (*i* was shown)—all possibilities of form in movement proceed from out of the universe, every possibility of movement that we out of the nature of our being are able to conceive and to bring into connection with the human organization.

My dear friends, one can indeed say that these possibilities of movement are those which, becoming fixed, give man his physical form as it is when he reaches full matuirty. What then would the gods do if they really wished to form man out of a lump of earth? The gods would make movements, and as a result of these movements, capable of giving form to the dust of the earth, the human form would eventually arise.

Now once more let us picture the eurythmy movements for *a*, for *b*, for *c*, and so on. Let us imagine that the gods, out of their divine primeval activity were to make those eurythmic movements which correspond to the sounds of the alphabet. Then, if these movements were impressed into physical matter, the human being would stand before us. This is what really lies behind eurythmy. The human being as we see him is a completed form. But the form has been created out of movement. It has arisen from those primeval forms which were continually taking shape and again passing away. Movement does not proceed from quiescence; on the contrary, that which is in a state of rest originates in movement. In eurythmy we are really going back to primordial movement.

What is it that my Creator, working out of primeval, cosmic being, does in me as man?

If you would give the answer to this question you must make the eurythmic movements. God eurythmetizes, and as the result of His eurythmy there arises the form of man.

36

What I have said here about eurythmy can indeed be said about any of the arts, for in some way or another every art springs from a divine origin. But in eurythmy most especially, because it makes use of the human being as its instrument, one is able to penetrate most deeply into the connection existing between the human being and the cosmic being. For this reason one cannot fail to appreciate eurythmy. For just suppose that one had no real conception of the nature of human beauty, as this is expressed in the outward human form, and then suppose that one had the opportunity of being shown how in the beginning, God created the beautiful human form out of movement, and one saw the repetition of those divine creative movements in the eurythmic gestures, then one would receive the answer to the question: How did human beauty come into being?

Let us think of the child, the incomplete human being, who has not yet attained to his full manhood. How shall we help the gods, so that the physical form of the child shall be rightly furthered in its development? What shall we bring to the child in the way of movement? We must teach him eurythmy, for this is a continuation of divine movement, of the divine creation of man.

And when illness of some kind or another overtakes the human being, then the forms corresponding to his divine archetype receive injury; here, in the physical world, they become different. What shall we do then? We must go back to those divine movements; we must help the sick human being to make those movements for himself. This will work upon him in such a way that the harm his bodily form may have received will be remedied.

Thus we have to look upon eurythmy as an art of healing, just as in ancient clairvoyant times it was known that certain sounds, uttered with a special intonation, re-acted upon the health of man. But in those days one was shown how to affect the health by a more or less roundabout way, by means of the air, which worked back again into the etheric body. If one works more directly, if one makes the patient actually do the movements corresponding to the formation of his

37

organs,—the point being, of course, that one knows what these movements really are,—(e.g., certain movements of the foot and leg correspond to certain formations right up in the head),—when one reproduces all this, then there arises this third aspect of eurythmy, curative eurythmy.

This introduction was necessary in order that all of you, as active eurythmists, may gain a fundamental feeling and perception of what you are doing. You must not take eurythmy as something which can be learned in the ordinary conventional way, but you must think of it as something which brings the human being nearer to the Divine than would otherwise be possible. The same applies indeed to all art. You must permeate yourselves through and through with this feeling. What then must be considered as an essential part of all eurythmic teaching? The right atmosphere must enter into it, the feeling for the connection between man and the divine spiritual powers. This is essential if you would become eurythmists in the true sense.

LECTURE 2

THE CHARACTER OF THE INDIVIDUAL SOUNDS

Dornach, 25th June 1924

Yesterday I attempted to portray the general character of speech as such and the character of this visible speech of eurythmy in particular. To-day I should like to describe the characteristics of the individual sounds, for only when the character and inner nature of these sounds reveal themselves to us shall we be able to understand the elements of eurythmy. To begin with I should like to draw attention to the fact that in the life of humanity, in the course of human evolution, there has always been a more or less definite consciousness of these things. It is only in our time that, as I said yesterday, we have become so shrivelled up with regard to our attitude towards speech. There has always existed a certain consciousness of all that lies in the progression of sounds as they occur in language, an understanding of the fact that in the consonants there lies an imitation of outer forms or outer happenings, and that an inward experience is contained in the vowel sounds.

This consciousness has been carried over more or less into the forms of the letters, so that in the formation of the letters in ancient languages, (in the Hebrew language for example, in the case of the consonants) we may still see a sort of imitation of what takes place in the air, of what forms itself in the air when we speak. To a great extent this has been lost in all the modern languages. (Among these I naturally include all those which, let us say, begin with the Latin language; the Greek language still retains something of what I mean.) Many things, however, still recall the time when attempts were made to imitate in the forming of the letters that which actually lies in the formation, in the structure of the word; when a word was fashioned out of the

39

consonantal element,—that is to say, the imitation of the external,—and out of the inner experience which had its source in the life of the soul. To-day it is only in certain interjections that we can still see clearly an instance of such imitation. Let us take an example which may serve to lead us more deeply into the real nature of eurythmy.

When we pronounce the sound *h*,—clearly, not merely as a breath,—we have a sound which really lies midway between the consonants and the vowels. This is always the case with sounds which have a special relation to breathing. Breathing was always felt to be something in which the human being lives partly in an inner experience and partly in an outgoing experience. Now the *h*-sound, this simple breath sound, may be felt,—and was indeed felt by primitive man,— as the imitation, the forming in the air of a *wafting process*, as the imitation of the way in which the breath is wafted into the surrounding atmosphere. Everything which is experienced as a wafting process is expressed through some word in which the *h*-sound is present, because the *h* itself is felt as the wafting process.

The vowel sound *u* can be felt as something which inwardly chills the soul, so that it takes on a certain rigidity and numbness. That is the inward experience lying behind *u*. *U* is the expression of something which chills, stiffens, benumbs; it is the sound which gives one the feeling of coldness. *U*, then, is the chilling, stiffening process.

And the *sch*,—that is the blowing away of something. It is the sound in which one feels that something is blowing past.

Now it is a fact that in certain districts, when an icy wind is blowing and one is numbed and stiff with the cold, people make use of the expression: husch-husch, husch-husch. In this interjection we still have an absolute experience of the *h-u-sch:* husch-husch. In primeval language all words were really interjections, ejaculations.

Let us take another combination of sounds. You all know the sound *r*. If one experiences the *r*-sound in the right way, one feels it as a turning wheel: *r-r-r-r.* Thus the *r* expresses a rolling, a revolving; it is the imitation of anything which gives the impression of turning, rolling, revolving. We must think of it, picture it, like this:

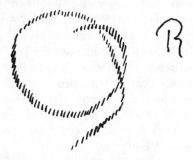

Yesterday I spoke already of the sound *a*. I told you that *a* expresses wonder. The *sch*-sound has already been described; it is the blowing past of something. And now we are able to feel the word ' rasch ' (swift). It is easy to picture it. When anything rushes past it creates a certain wonder and disappears, is blown away: *rasch*.

So you see there is a good reason for regarding the consonants as being an imitation. Here we have in the *r* the revolving, rolling, turning of something; in the vowel-sound *a* the inner feeling of wonder: in the *sch*-sound something which goes away, which passes by.

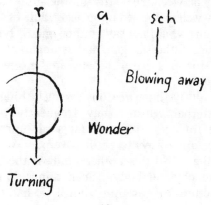

From these examples you can already see that there is a certain justification for speaking of a primeval language, for you can feel that if human beings really experienced the sounds absolutely truly they would all speak in the same way; they would quite naturally, out of their own organization, describe things exactly in the same way.

It is a fact, as Spiritual Science teaches us, that there was once upon the earth a primeval language. You all know myths and legends dealing with this,—but it is much more than a myth or a legend. There is really something which lies at the back of all languages, and which is, in the way I have described, the primeval language from which all other languages have been built up.

When one turns one's attention to certain facts of life and sees how, out of an infinite wisdom, they have been given similar names, then one is quite overwhelmed with the wisdom which reigns in the whole evolution of man, indeed in the whole evolution of the world. Consider the following, my dear friends,—and what I am now going to bring forward is no mere triviality—it rests on an actual primal sense in man.

For people who think deeply over the problems which present themselves to the understanding, certain things that bear somewhat intimate relationship to life itself become riddles,—riddles which are simply passed over by the more blunted sensibilities of the average man. The fact that there is a similarity between the words 'mother-milk' and 'mother-tongue' may well be looked upon as a riddle of this kind. It is clear that one would not say 'father-milk', but the reason for not saying 'father-tongue' is less apparent. Where are we to seek for this parallel between 'mother-milk' and 'mother-tongue'?

There are always inner reasons for such things. It is true that the external reasons may frequently be brilliantly proved, but for these intimate facts of human evolution inner reasons are always to be discovered. When the child comes into the world the mother's milk is the best nourishment for the physical body. Such things do not properly belong to lectures on eurythmy, but if we had the necessary

42

time, and if we were to analyse the mother's milk in the right way,—not with the dead methods of chemistry but with a living chemistry,—we should find out why it is that the mother's milk is the best nourishment for the physical body of man during the first stages of life.—Indeed, speaking from the medical-scientific point of view, one may go so far as to say that the milk of the mother is the best means of building up, of actually giving form to the physical body. This is the first thing we have to realize. It is the mother's milk which gives form to the physical body. And it is the " mother-tongue ',—we said yesterday that the mother-tongue corresponds to the etheric body,—it is the mother-tongue which develops and gives form to the etheric body. For this reason we have a similarity between the words. First there appears the physical body with its need for the mother's milk and then the etheric body with its need for the mother-tongue.

A deep wisdom lies hidden in such things. We find the deepest wisdom, not only in these word formations which can be traced back to ancient times, but also in many proverbial sayings and ideas. We should not look upon the wisdom concealed in old sayings and proverbs merely as superstition, but should recognize that very often wonderful and significant traditions are contained within them.

Having said this, having made my meaning clear to you, let us now proceed to a description of the nature of the sounds. When we understand what the sounds represent, how the vowels are the expression of inward experiences and the consonants the imitation of the external world,—when we understand how this is the case in every single instance,— then we are led to a threefold study of eurythmy,—artistic, educational and curative. I shall make use of everything which could possibly serve to give you a vivid picture of the individual sounds as they really are, so that to-morrow you will be able fully to understand the plastic gestures which we make use of in eurythmy.

In *a* there lies a feeling of wonder, astonishment. In *b*, as I told you yesterday, we have the imitation of something which protects and shelters us from what is outside ourselves. In *b* we feel that we are enveloped in something. This can even be seen in the way that the letter is formed, only in modern writing the sheath is, as it were, doubled: *B*. *B* is always an enveloping, a kind of shelter. To put it somewhat crudely *b* might be said to be the house in which one lives. *B* is a house.

In my characterization of the various sounds in speech-eurythmy I shall take the German language as my starting point. I could just as easily take the sounds of more ancient languages, but we will make a beginning with the German sounds and see how these reveal themselves to us in their true nature.*

Coming now to the sound *c* (ts),—I shall naturally not go into the formation of the written letters as these have mostly become degenerate and in any case, eurythmists do not need to interest themselves so much in language from this point of view,—coming now to the sound *c* you will feel it to be something which is in movement. It would be impossible to feel that with the sound *c* one would try to imitate anything which is in a state of rest. There is a certain impact in the sound *c*; nevertheless, when you really experience what lies behind it, you will realize how impossible it would be to picture anything heavy in connection with it. It would never occur to you that with *c* you would wish to imitate something which would make you get into a great heat if you tried to lift it. On the contrary, the feeling that one has is that here is the imitation of something which is the reverse of heavy, which is really very light. It is the quality of lightness that is really imitated in the sound *c*. Thus one can say quite simply: In *c* we have the imitation of *lightness*.

If you enter into the intimate nature of the different sounds, you will, in the case of *c*, have much the same feeling as if in a circus you saw weights,—apparently made of iron and marked so and so many hundredweight,—lifted up quickly and easily by the clown. Imagine that you were to approach such a weight, in the belief that it were made of iron

* See footnote on page 28

44

and immensely heavy, and that you were to lift it up. You would approach it, and in suddenly raising it, you would produce a movement very similar to the sound *c*. We have the same thing in Nature; for sneezing is not all at unlike a *c*. Sneezing is a lightening process.

It was said by the old occultists that the sound *c* in primeval language was the Regent of Health. And in Austria, when a person sneezes, we still have a saying: *Zur Gesundheit* (Your very good health). These are feelings which must be taken into consideration when studying the sounds, otherwise we shall not be able to come to any understanding of them in their reality.

D,—when should we be most naturally wishing to use the sound *d*? *d. d. d.* If someone were to ask you where a thing was, and you knew, the movement you would make to show him,—you can feel it—would be best accompanied by the sound *d*. And if you wished to indicate that you expected your questioner to be astonished at getting such a speedy answer, then you would say: *da* (there). If you leave out the astonishment, the wonder, then there remains just the *d*. In such a case you are not so conceited as to wish to call up in your questioner the feeling of wonder; you simply show him where the thing is. In expressing *d* one makes what may be called indicating movements raying out in all directions. It is not difficult to feel this. So that we may say: *D* is the *pointing towards something*, the *raying out towards something*. The imitation of this pointing, of this raying out, of this drawing attention to something, all this lies in the sound *d*.

E is a sound which has always been of very special interest. As you already know *e* is the sound which gives expression to the feeling that something has been done to us and we stand up against it. *E: we will not allow what has been done to trouble us.*

Here it may be well to introduce the sound *t*, *Tao*, and to explain its significance. You are perhaps already aware that a deep reverence rises up in those who begin to understand what lies in this sound. This *Tao*, *t*, is really the sound

45

which has to be felt as representing something of the greatest importance. We may even go so far as to say that it contains within it creative forces, forces which also have a radiating, indicating quality, but with *t* it is more especially a radiance which streams from heaven down on to the earth. There is a weightiness about the sound, and at the same time also a radiance. Thus we can say: *T* is *the streaming of forces from above downwards.*

Now it is, of course, possible for something which under certain conditions has to be felt as having great and majestic qualities also to make its appearance in ordinary everyday life. Let us take three sounds. Let us first take *e* as we have learned to know it. *E* expresses the feeling: Something has been done to me, but I stand up against it and assert myself. *T, Tao:* Something has burst in upon me. Let us try to show what is contained in this experience: Something has been done to me but I stand up against it—*e*. An event has taken place; it has suddenly burst in upon me—*t*: but it is soon over, it passes over; the blowing away of something—*sch*. In this way we get the following combination of sounds: *etsch*. When do we make use of this expression? We use it when, for instance, somebody makes an important statement, which is, however, false, and we immediately jump to the conclusion that it *is* false. Now when we are in a position immediately to get rid of what has affected us, when this statement or whatever it is has burst in upon us like a flash of lightning but we destroy it and blow it away, then we say: *etsch*. Here you have an explanation of this combination of sounds. One feels the *e* particularly strongly, the being affected by something. One could not imagine saying *itsch* or *atsch* in such a case. But in an experience of this kind, when one has been affected by something but has been able immediately to get rid of it, then one obviously must use the expression: *etsch*.

Now out of the way in which you form the movement for *e*, out of your knowledge of eurythmy, you will be able fully to enter into the gesture that in many districts accompanies this expression. This gesture is really very similar to the eurythmic movement for *e*.   *Etsch, etsch* (showing the corresponding movement).   Here we actually have the eurythmic movement for *e*.   Such movements are absolutely natural and instinctive.

Thus behind the sound *e* there lies the experience of being affected by something and of withstanding it.   Naturally when one describes such things the description tends to be awkward and inadequate.   Everything   depends on being able to feel what is meant.

F is a sound which is somewhat difficult to experience in an age which has such a lifeless, dried-up conception of language.   But it may perhaps be of assistance to us, my dear friends, if I remind you of a phrase which you all know and which is in fairly general use.   People say, when somebody knows a thing upside down and inside out: Er kennt die Sache aus dem *ff*.   (He knows it out of the *ff*.)   An extraordinarily interesting experience lies behind this phrase. When one finds the man in the street making use of such an expression and compares it with what was said in the old Mysteries the result is truly remarkable.   (You remember I said that I should make use of everything which could help us to gain a true understanding of the sounds, whether my examples were drawn from a cultured or from a more primitive source,—the latter being the more fruitful, naturally.) In the ancient Mysteries there was still a living understanding of the words: ' In the beginning was the Word, and the Word was with God '; there was still a living feeling for the creative power of the Word, of the Logos.   (Logos is not to be translated ' wisdom '; indeed, by doing so many modern scholars have betrayed their lack of understanding for these things.   Logos must unquestionably be translated ' Verbum', ' Word ',—only the word ' Word ' must be understood in the right way, in the way in which I explained it yesterday.) Now, in the old Mysteries of Western Asia, Southern Asia and Africa it was said, when speaking about the sound *f*: When man utters the sound *f* he expels out of himself the whole stream of his breath.   It was by means of the breath that the Gods created man, and the whole of human wisdom

47

is contained in the air, in the breath. So that all the Indian was able to learn when through Yoga Philosophy he learned to control his breathing and as a result was able to fill himself with inner wisdom,—all this he felt when he uttered the sound *f*. In the old Indian Yoga practices the pupil had the following experience: he practised Yoga exercises, the technique of which consisted in this, that he became inwardly aware of the organization of man, inwardly aware of the fullness of wisdom. In uttering the sound *f* he became conscious of the wisdom contained in the Word. *F* can therefore only be rightly understood when one tries even to-day to understand a certain formula, which is very little known in the world, but which nevertheless did once exist and in the old Egyptian Mysteries ran somewhat as follows: *If thou wouldst proclaim the nature of Isis, of Isis who contains within herself the knowledge of the past, present and future and from whom the veil can never entirely be lifted, then thou must do this in the sound f.*

The making use of the process of breathing in order to fill oneself with the being of Isis, the experiencing of Isis in the out-going breath-stream,—this it is that lies in the sound *f*. So that *f*—not indeed exactly, but at any rate to some extent —can be felt as the expression of: I know.—But more lies in it than this. ' I know ' is really only a feeble expression of what we should feel in the sound *f*. For this very reason the feeling for *f* was soonest lost. *F* may be felt somewhat as follows: Know thou, to whom I speak, when I say *f* to thee I would make thee aware that I can teach thee. Thou must know that I myself have knowledge.—

It would therefore seem natural to you, absolutely natural, if someone desirous of putting another right were suddenly to approach him giving vent to a sound similar to *f*. There are many interesting words, words which would well repay study, in which the sound *f* occurs in some connection or other. This study, however, you can carry out for yourselves; and you will be reminded of all that I have told you about the inner nature of the sound *f*.

I have already spoken about the sound *h*; we know that it is the blowing, the wafting past of something.

And now *i*. It is easy to feel *i* as an *assertion of oneself*, as positive self-assertion. In the German language there is a very happy example of this. It is our word for the expression of the affirmation or the assertion of something: Ja (yes). Here certainly there is the indication of a consonantal element, but the *i* is nevertheless present and is followed by wonder, by amazement. Assent, affirmation, cannot be better expressed than by assertion of self coloured by wonder. We said yesterday that the quality of wonder really represented man in his true being; and when we add to this the assertion of oneself: Ja,—then we could not have a clearer, more definite expression of the affirmative. Thus in *i* we have the assertion of self. We shall see how important it is for eurythmists to understand that behind the sound *i* there is always a vindication of oneself, an assertion of oneself.

L is a very remarkable sound,—as I am pronouncing it now it contains a hint of *e*,—but I mean the pure sound *l*. Try to realize what you really do when you pronounce *l*. Try to realize especially what you do with your tongue. You use your tongue in a very skilful way when you pronounce the sound *l*. *l*, *l*, *l*. You become aware of a creative, form-giving element when saying this sound. Indeed, if one were not too terribly hungry, one might almost satisfy one's hunger by simply saying the sound *l* very distinctly and over and over again. We feel *l* to be something absolutely real, as real, for example, as if we were to eat a dumpling—a specially nice, soft dumpling—and were to allow it to melt on the tongue with a feeling of great satisfaction. We can have a like experience when we pronounce the sound *l*, *l*, *l*, very distinctly. There is something creative, something form-giving in this sound. And the sculptor is very much tempted when working on the figures which he is creating to make a movement of the tongue similar to the movement which the tongue makes when forming the sound *l*. Though of course the sculptor does not say *l* aloud; he only makes a similar movement with his tongue. And anyone able to feel the shape of a nose, for instance, with his tongue,—where the feeling for form, the feeling of *l* is so strong,—such a one

49

would undoubtedly be very successful in modelling noses! It was said in the old Mysteries that *l* is the creative, form-giving element in all things and beings,—*the force which overcomes matter in the creation of form.*

You will easily feel that the diphthong *ei** corresponds to an affectionate caress. When dealing with a child one often makes use of this sound. *Ei, ei—an affectionate caress.*

I shall next have to describe the sound *m*, and we shall see that *m* has the quality of entering right into something, of taking on the form of something outside itself. Let us now suppose, my dear friends,—and here again I am not merely trifling but what I have to say is drawn from out of the history of the ages,—let us suppose that we had some sort of substance and assume that this substance should be the means of transforming matter, of giving form to matter. Let us put the story together. In the first place we demand of this substance that it shall transform matter and give it form and shape. That is to be its main attribute. It is to give form to matter, but in such a way that it clings closely and lovingly to something other than itself, in much the same way as when one caresses a little child: *ei, ei,*—this is the expression of a caressing quality. The substance must cling to something. And this clinging quality must be retained; the substance must as it were take on a form which is foreign to it, so that it appears exactly the same as this external form; it imitates this form quite exactly. And now let us suppose that we express this transformation of matter into form by means of a combination of sounds. We say *l*. The clinging quality, *ei*. The taking on of some external form: *m*. Thus we have a word: *Leim* (glue) which is quite specially characteristic in the German language, quite apart from any other consideration. It is upon such combinations of sound behind which there lies hidden the active, evolving genius of language, that the *life* of this genius of language really depends. It occurs from time to time that when in some language or other a word already exists, although perhaps in a vague, indefinite form, that this word is metamorphosed and

* German *ei*, English *i* (as in sight).

50

introduced again into a language of a later development, retaining a similarity to its original feeling if the nation which receives it has a sense for it.　An understanding of language is a much more complicated matter than is usually supposed. To-day people treat language in a really terrible fashion. In ordinary everyday life which rests upon superficiality and convention such a treatment of language is perhaps not out of place; but its effect upon the human soul is nothing short of devastating, *how* utterly devastating it is impossible to say.　For instance, somebody wishes to translate a book or a poem.　So he proceeds to hunt in the dictionary or to search his memory in order to discover the corresponding words.　And having more or less transposed it in this way he calls it a translation.　But it would really be more correct to call it a *mis-translation*,—for this is a wrong track altogether.　Nothing is more appalling than this method of transferring something from one language into another.

Let us therefore study this question from the following point of view.　Assuming that there was once a primeval language (alike of course for all men),—and there is no doubt that this language did exist,—assuming that there was once a primeval language, then the question naturally arises: How is it that the many different languages came into being? How does it come about that if we take a German word, the word ' Kopf ' (head) for instance, and translate this into Italian, we have to say ' testa '?　We have the German word ' Kopf ' and the Italian word: ' testa '.　When we begin to enter into the true nature of language we must ask ourselves the question: How is it that the Italian feels the sounds in ' testa ' which are totally different from those felt by the German when he makes use of the word: ' Kopf '?　According to the rules of translation the two words should have the same significance.　If the word ' Kopf ' were really to be experienced, then the Italian, and even the Chinese would perforce have to say ' Kopf ' also.　How then can the origin of the different languages be explained.

What I am now going to say may make you double up with

laughter, but it is nevertheless true. The German makes use of the word 'Kopf'; the Italian would also make use of this word if he wished to designate the same thing. But he does not wish to do so. The German point of view lies outside his field of vision. What the German expresses in the word 'Kopf', that to which he gives the name 'Kopf' does not occur in the vocabulary of the Italian language. Were the Italian desirous of expressing the same thing, he, like the German, would say: 'Kopf'. What then does the German mean when he says: 'Kopf'? He means to describe the *form*, the rounded form of the head. It is easy to feel this rounded form in the word 'Kopf'. Later on when we have studied the sound *k* and all that we need in this connection, we shall be able to realize more clearly that it is the rounded form which is meant here. Now when the word 'Kopf' is shown in eurythmy try to see how this rounding appears in the middle of the word. (Demonstration). The German describes as 'Kopf' the round form of the head as it rests on the shoulders.

Were the Italian to have the same experience, he also would say: 'Kopf' not: 'testa'. What then does he experience? The Italian does not experience the rounded form, but he feels what is implied in a statement, in a testimony; he is more aware of what underlies the word '*testament*'. Thus the act of making a testimony, making a declaration, an affirmation, this it is which is felt by the Italian and for this reason he says: 'testa'. He means something totally different from the German. The words 'Kopf' and 'testa' only appear to describe the same thing; in reality they are fundamentally different. In the one case, in the German word, the form of the head is described as it rests upon the shoulders. And in German, if one wishes to lay emphasis upon the roundness of the form one can make use of an expression which has in it at the same time a certain element of contempt and say: 'Kohlkopf'. (Cabbage-head. Block-head.) You will agree with me that here there can be no shadow of doubt that the rounded form is meant.

But the head as it rests upon the shoulders is not felt as a round form by the Italian; he feels it to be something which makes an assertion, a declaration. For this reason he says: ' testa ', and feels in this word all that I have described.

This lack of understanding is very general among translators. As a rule we translate without paying any attention to the fact that we should transpose ourselves into the whole atmosphere of the other language in order to catch its exact shades of meaning. Just think how external it is when one translates according to a dictionary. One misses just those things which are most essential and passes them by in sublime unconsciousness.

Let us now return to the sound *m*,—that sound which makes such a wonderful ending to the sacred Indian word *Aum*. *M* contains within it the element of comprehension, of understanding. In the way in which the sound is carried on the stream of the breath we feel that it *conforms itself to everything and understands everything*. *M* signifies that which is deeply felt and understood. I remember that my village schoolmaster said *mhn* when he wanted to show that I had answered a question rightly. At such times he always said *mhn*,—i.e. he understood it, he agreed with it; the *hn* was only the expression of his satisfaction. *M*, therefore, may be said to be the expression of agreement. It clings to some thing and is in agreement with it, as the *m* at the end of the word *Leim*.

It is clear from these few examples that in each sound there lies concealed a whole world of experience. And we can easily realize that if we were to express ourselves by means of sounds only, instead of using our ordinary words, we should indeed have a simpler and more primitive language, but it would be one which would combine with this simplicity a much deeper intimacy and understanding.

As eurythmists it is very necessary that you should gradually feel your way into the real nature of the sounds; for eurythmy does indeed consist of a plastic formation of movement and gesture. Such movements are, however, in no way arbitrary nor transient. On the contrary the move-

53

ments of eurythmy are cosmic in their nature, they are full of significance, they could in no way be other than they are.

In the next lecture I shall describe to you the other sounds which I have not touched upon to-day, and then gradually we shall consider the main characteristics of the actual movements which we use in eurythmy. We shall see how these movements express in their very essence exactly the same as is expressed by the sounds themselves as they are breathed into the air, as they take shape in the air.

a: Wonder
Amazement
b: To wrap round; to envelop
c: (ts) The quality of lightness
d: To indicate; to ray outwards
e: To be affected by something and to withstand it
t: A significant streaming from above downwards
f: Thou knowest that I know
i: Assertion of self
l: The overcoming of matter by form
m: To be in agreement

husch
husch!
{ h: The wafting breath sound
u: The becoming chilled and stiffened
sch: The blowing past of something

Rasch
{ r: Rolling, revolving
a: Wonder
sch: Blowing past

Leim
{ l: The transforming of matter into form
ei: The quality of clinging
m: Imitation, combined with understanding

LECTURE 3

THE GESTURES; HOW THEY ARE FORMED AND EXPERIENCED

Dornach, 26th June 1924

To-day it is my intention to describe those sounds which have not yet been considered. To begin with I shall take *s* and *z*, for the nature of these sounds is such that they may almost be said to be in a category by themselves. Later, as opportunity arises, I can deal with any of the sounds which up to now have been omitted.

S was always felt, at a time when such things had not yet been lost, as a sound penetrating specially deeply into the very essence of language. The experience of the *s*-sound is connected with the feelings and experiences which, in the earliest times of human evolution, were bound up with the symbol of the serpent, and also, from a certain point of view, with the symbol of the Staff of Mercury,—not with the symbol of Mercury itself, but with the symbol of the Staff of Mercury. We must look for the Mercury symbol itself in the sound *e*. On the other hand the symbol of the Staff of Mercury, which plays so great a part in certain Eastern writings, is very closely connected with the sound *s*; and the *s*-form which we still preserve to-day in our written letter reminds us strongly of the symbol of the serpent. The feeling lying behind the curved and sinuous line of *s* is really extraordinarily complicated, but primarily it may be said to consist of a powerful peace-bringing element, bringing calm and peace into that which is in a state of unrest, and this force carries with it the feeling of certainty, *the feeling of being able to penetrate into the hidden nature of something and in so doing to bring about a state of calmness and rest.*

The *S*-symbol, and the *z* which is closely related to it, were always referred to in the Mysteries with great solemnity. Such things, as we saw yesterday when studying the sound *t*,

55

Tao, were always spoken of with a fitting ceremony and reverence. *S*, on the other hand,—and here I am bound to express myself very inadequately,—*s* always produced an element of fear in those who were being instructed in the nature of this symbol. There was a feeling of fear; it was felt as something to be guarded against, but which was nevertheless essential to life, something which could not be dispensed with. I cannot easily tell you how it was spoken of in the Mysteries. The most I can do is to try and describe it for you in other words.

People to-day would be astonished if they could know how entirely free from sentimentality the true pupils of the old Mysteries really were. They had a sense of humour and although none knew better than they how to pay reverence where reverence was due, they knew also how to clothe such things in humoristic form. Thus, when a pupil of the Mysteries was asked by one not initiated about the nature of the sound *s*—(naturally such questions were often asked, for people of those earlier times were not without curiosity any more than they are now)—when this question was put, the pupil replied somewhat humorously: Well, you know, when one understands the secret of the *s*-sound, then one can perceive the hidden qualities in the hearts of men and one can fathom the hearts of women: such a one can bring calm to the restlessness of the human heart, and can at the same time penetrate into its hidden depths.—That was, as I said, a very exoteric explanation, but it nevertheless gives some indication of what lies in the sound *s*. *S*—a bringing of calm into that which is agitated, and the certainty that the means employed will have the desired effect.

When all that I have just described is carried over into gesture, then we get the eurythmic movement for the sound *s*. We have still to consider the sound *z*, and the feeling, the experience, that it expresses. The movement for *z* is naturally somewhat similar to the movement for *c* (ts), but with more of an attack behind it. You will be able to feel for yourselves, if you try to do so with the necessary earnestness and enthusiasm, that this sound induces a certain feeling of

56

gaiety, for the very reason that it is not heavy and can be taken lightly; it is, however, gay with a certain intention. This can, of course, apply also to an inanimate object.

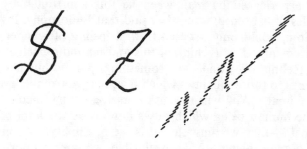

Now we have realized to some extent the meaning of most of the sounds, and have reached a point at which it should be possible for each individual sound to call up in our souls a corresponding experience. I said earlier that these first lectures were to be in the nature of a recapitulation in order to establish a tradition which may be regarded as permanent. Now once again let us call up in our minds each separate sound in its eurythmic significance.

It is above all things important that everything I have said about the nature of the various sounds should be experienced artistically as gesture.

There is one thing about which we must be quite clear; the human being is formed out of those cosmic elements which I have mentioned in connection with the sounds of speech. If you take all that we have connected with these sounds, you will get, roughly speaking, in a perfectly natural way, those impulses which lead the human being out of the pre-earthly existence into earthly existence, and which guide him further until he reaches mature age, that is to say until about his thirty-fifth year.

This whole process, with the forces which separate, which urge him forward and bring him to the point he finally reaches as an adult human being,—all this lies in the gestures expressing the sounds. That is why the Word, the spoken sound, was felt as of such tremendous significance.

57

Now let us begin by referring once more to that quality which is most intimately bound up with the human being, and which was described by the Greeks when they said that it was experienced by man when he was confronted by the riddles of existence, when they said that Philosophy, love of wisdom, could only proceed from a feeling of wonder and amazement. Let us think of this and remind ourselves that the feeling of wonder is something purely human and belongs to those qualities which raise man above the level of the animal. And when we ask ourselves: What faculty is it in the human being which raises him above the level of the animal?—then we must say: It is the possibility, inherent in the human being, to keep flexible, certain proportions, forces or rather, directions of forces, which in the realm of animals have been forced into strict forms. Man must therefore be looked upon as a centre towards which certain forces gravitate and in which they are finally merged. There would be a sense of monotony in the idea that the origin of man, which should call up in him a feeling of wonder and awe, must be looked for as proceeding from one single point of the universe,—which is indeed the case with the plants and the animals. That which calls up in man the feeling of wonder with regard to his own being can only be felt by him as coming from different directions of cosmic space. And we only understand ourselves as men, in our true human dignity when we begin to realize that the Gods are radiating their forces into us from the surrounding cosmos.

Let us make some sort of diagram of the cosmic sphere (see drawing) showing how forces are streaming from the circumference towards the centre, towards the earth (arrows).

We can only feel our own dignity as human beings on the earth when we understand how these forces are flowing into us from out of the different directions of the cosmos.

Make the eurythmic movement for *a*. The fundamental nature of this movement lies in the fact that you reach out, as it were, with your hands and arms into two different directions of space. *A* does not really consist in making a free, swinging movement, but one has to imagine oneself as man

58

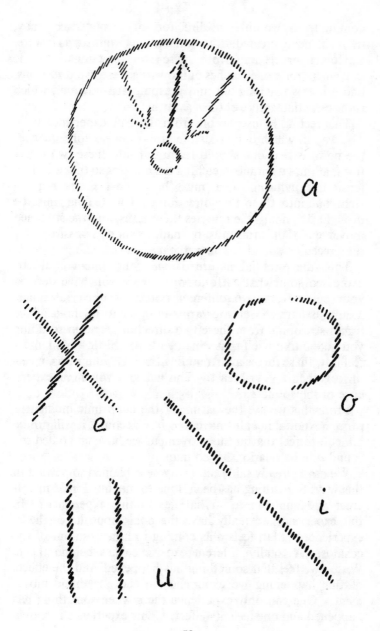

coming from two different directions of cosmic space,—nay, more, as being created, differentiated, determined, as it were, by forces proceeding from these two directions. In the movement for *a* one reaches out towards these two directions, and it is this reaching out and grasping at something which is the essential feature of the *a* as such.

This feeling is inseparable from the true experience of *a*. The way in which one holds the arms is of no consequence; the point is that one should reach out into these two directions, at the same time stretching the muscles so that a certain tension is induced. One must have the feeling of going right out into these two directions. This feeling must be brought down into the muscles themselves, and the stretched movement of the arms must be made as soon as possible after the preceding sound. This is the *a* as such.

Thus the essential nature of the *a*-movement could be expressed somewhat as follows: O man, you have derived your being from two different points of universal space. You must stretch out your arms in order to lay hold of the forces streaming from these two directions, and in so doing you take into ourself that which gave you birth. You must feel how these forces are streaming through your arms, meeting together in your breast. This will give you a real experience of the sound *a*.

From this we see the nature of the eurythmic movement for *a*. And taking all I have said into account, it will not be difficult to feel that in this movement we have embodied the sound *a* in its relationship to man.

We have already said that *e* may be explained somewhat in this way: Something has been done to me, but I hold myself erect and confront it. What lies in this experience? In this experience we really have the polar opposite of the *a*-experience. Man feels *a* as coming to him from out of the cosmos. A totally different experience lies behind the *e*. With *e* we feel that something has happened, and the effects of this happening we experience in the eurythmic movement. One can only experience the *e* when something has happened and one feels its effect. This experience is shown in the movement *when one part of the organism is brought into direct contact with another part.*

Now this cannot be done in very many ways. Man is differently built from the elephant, for instance, and is therefore not able to make his nose so long and flexible that with its tip he could touch his own back. Were he able to do this it would be a most excellent example of the movement for, *e.* He cannot do it, however. And so the movement for *e*, as it occurs in our eurythmy, can only be made by one limb actually touching the other, laying a certain emphasis on this contact. This at the same time expresses the feeling of *confronting something and resisting it.* The touching indicates the feeling that something has happened to one; the holding the position which must be in the nature of two crossed lines, corresponds to the feeling of resistance. With *e* one arm is laid upon the other; or one finger can be laid upon the other; or the possibility exists, if one is able to manage it, of so using the eyes that the direction of the gaze of one eye crosses the direction of the gaze of the other. Any movement, therefore, in which this experience of touching one part of the organism with another is really present, may be said to be the eurythmic expression for the sound *e*. When, however, the gesture is held fast, thus showing that something has been done to one and one gathers one's forces together in order to withstand it, then the complete experience is brought to visible expression. Just consider what an immense difference there is between the *a* and the *e*-sounds as these are expressed in the movements of eurythmy.

The *a*-experience carries with it the necessity of a conscious stretching of the muscles. It is essential that you really feel this tension. The *e*-experience carries with it the necessity of resting one arm upon the other; and here the consciousness should mainly be centred at the point where the arms cross.

Thus it is not the stretching of the muscles which is the chief thing about the experience of the *e*-sound, but the resting, the pressing of one arm upon the other. Of course it is also possible to form the *e* by crossing the right leg over the left, at the same time pressing one against the other. In this way we experience the *e*, we feel the movement for *e*.

Now, in our modern civilization one may easily get the impression that the world is always 'doing something' to people, is always affecting them, for they usually sit with crossed legs, and by so doing are of course continually making the movement for *e*! This attitude betrays the fact that the great majority of people believe that the world has indeed done something to them and that they must stand up against it. Thus does it appear to an artistic approach in the sphere of gesture.

When we now pass on to the movement for *o*, to the gesture for *o*, we shall feel what a world of experience is contained in this sound. *A* is the absolute expression of wonder and amazement. *O* expresses the feeling which we have when we place ourselves in an intelligent relationship to something which at the same time calls forth our wonder. And indeed, if we are human beings in the true sense, everything which enters into our field of vision must call up in us a feeling of wonder. But *o* brings us into a more intimate relationship with our perceptions. So that the essential nature of *o* can be shown in eurythmy when the human being does not only feel himself, but, going out from himself, feels some other being or object which he wishes to embrace.

You can most clearly get a picture of this when, out of love for another person, you put your arms around him. You get the absolutely natural movement for the sound *o* when, in embracing another person, the arms are rounded and bent, each taking on the form of a half-circle.

Thus, in the movement for *a*, we feel that we receive something. We reach out towards those regions of the cosmos from which man derives his being. In the *e* we have an indication of a direct experience. The human being experiences something coming from the outer world. In *o* we have the movement whereby the world experiences something through man himself, for in this movement man lays hold of something belonging to the outer world. You must try to make the movement for *o* in such a way that, from the very beginning, and right through to the very end, the arms are really rounded. The arms must be very flexible; they must really be rounded. This is the true movement for *o*. We have to feel the rounded form from the very beginning.

Now we come to that sound which is still clearer to man than the sound *e*,—we come to that sound which is the absolute expression of the assertion of self, that is to say the *i*-sound. *I* is self-assertion pure and simple. I have often drawn attention to the fact that in the every-day speech of educated people we find the word ' ich ' (I). In this word we have the feeling of self-assertion as expressed in the *i*, and to this is added a breath-sound (ch) whereby an indication is given that we, as human beings, live in the breathing. But in certain districts where the simple people speak in dialect, things are not carried so far as this. Such people remain satisfied with plain, straight-forward self-assertion. For this reason, in the place where I was brought up, people said, for instance, not 'ich', but ' i '. There it would have occurred to nobody to say ' Ich haue dich durch ' (I will give you a jolly good thrashing);—this expression occurs to me because in the place where I grew up one heard it on all sides, and because, with certain people, it really sums up their conception of the ego:—in my birthplace people do not say ' Ich haue dich durch ', but ' I hau di durch '! Pure self-assertion! This is a real example of pure self-assertion. Now, as we know, with *a*, forces stream from two points of the circumference inwards; with *i* they stream from the centre outwards. With the *i*-sound we do not feel as if we are grasping at something, but we feel the stretching, we feel that the stream has its source in us, starting as it were, from the heart and flowing through the arm, or through both arms, or through the legs. We can also feel *i* with the eyes, when we consciously look more through one eye, leaving the other passive. This gives us a very definite feeling of *i*.

There is nothing of the *a*-character about *i*, but both the arms should as a rule be used in such a way that one is the continuation of the other, although of course we can also

63

make use of one arm only. The chief thing to remember is that with *i* the main feeling must be that of stretching, whereas with *a* there is more the feeling of grasping at something. These nuances are of importance if we are to lay the right emphasis upon the individual sounds.

It is only when such shades of feeling are brought into the sounds of speech,—and indeed into the tones of music also, as I made clear in the course of lectures on tone-eurythmy which I gave here recently,—it is only then that eurythmy becomes truly artistic. The point is not so much, my dear friends, that you merely *imitate* the form, but that you inwardly *experience* the form; that is to say you must really get the feeling in both your arms that *a* is the *taking hold* of something which comes towards you, while you must feel *i* as a *stretched movement*, as a stretching out away from yourself.

Then again we have the *u*-sound about which I have already spoken. *U* is not the assertion of self; on the contrary, behind *u* there is the feeling of becoming smaller, of being chilled and stiffened with cold. There is the feeling of drawing back into oneself, of holding fast to oneself. Whereas with the sound *e* the principal thing is that one limb touches another at a single point with *u* the principal feeling is one of holding back.

The *u* is most clearly expressed by holding the arms as near together as possible, but this need only be indicated. There need only be an indication of this pressing together of the arms. When we stand with our legs together, touching one another, we are also expressing the sound *u*. And, as we have already seen, such movements can be made backwards as well as forwards.

Ei,—the *ei*-sound can best be felt—and this will throw light on what I said already yesterday—when one realizes that behind this sound there lies the same caressing, affectionate feeling that one has for a very little child: *ei, ei*,—it is as if one were stroking something, as if one were becoming intimate with something through one's feeling. (Frau L. . . . will show us a beautiful *e-i*.) Hold the body quite still; do not move the body in any way, but hold it quite still. You

64

will notice at once that in this gesture there is expressed the feeling of becoming intimate with something, but you will notice at the same time that our manner of writing, the way in which (in the German language), we form the *ei* out of the *e-i*, does not naturally lie in the *ei*-sound itself. On the contrary the *ei*-sound must be felt as a unity. We enter into the nature of *ei* when we join together *e* and *i*, but in fact *ei* lies midway between the two, and the connection between them is not really organic. I shall speak later about the more subtle nuances of feeling lying in this sound.

Let us now proceed to the consonants, and let us try to feel the consonantal element as this comes to expression in the movements. You will remember that I said: *b* is the sound which represents everything of an enveloping nature, it expresses the wrapping round of something and its corresponding movement is one of protection. Naturally the gesture as such does not express this fully; there must also be the actual experience of which the movement is the copy, is the imitation. (We will ask Frau F. . . . to show us the movement.) Now we have the true movement for *b*; let us hold it fast.

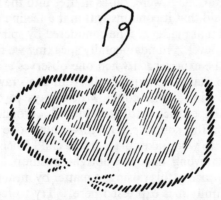

Thus we have the true movement for *b*, and in this movement we feel what really lies behind the position of each arm. Anyone experiencing what is contained in this movement might well say: I will picture to myself that I have something

65

before me, something that I wish to take hold of,—let us say a little child. I will imagine that I have such a little child sitting before me and that I wish to take it up. I shall be able to do this most easily when I take hold of it so, drawing it to me with a protecting gesture (movement for *b*).—What then must one really feel here if one would have the true experience? One must really feel that one holds something —here, in the space enclosed by the arms. If at this juncture I may introduce a point of educational interest, I would say that the best way to make the sound *b* comprehensible to small children in the eurythmy lesson is to take something or other and let the child clasp it in its arms. In this way you can teach the little child to understand that it should feel that its arms are the protecting shelter for the animal or object which it holds, and in this way it will learn fully to comprehend the nature of the *b*-movement.

All this is really essential to eurythmy. The forms, the movements, must not be imitated in a purely abstract manner, but the corresponding experiences must be felt; the experience is inseparable from the movement.

Now, I told you yesterday that *c* (ts) is a specially interesting sound. *C*, as it were, raises matter into the realm of the spirit. I said that it contains within it a feeling of lightness; it indicates that matter can be conquered by spirit and raised to a higher level. Fundamentally speaking we may say that *c* can best be experienced when one observes a child who is learning to stand, to raise itself from the crawling to the upright position. One could wish always to connect this wonderful experience—(for it is indeed a wonderful experience)—with the sound *c*. In this sound one approaches very nearly to what takes place in the child when it lifts itself from the crawling into the upright position, *c*, *c*, *c*: this lightening process, this raising of matter by means of spirit,— how beautifully it is expressed here! Try to feel all this in the sound *c*; feel that it has a lightness, that matter is raised up by means of spirit. You will most easily have the right feeling for the movement *c* when you imagine that in some inexplicable way something is lying on the surface of your

66

arms and in making the movement you toss it upwards. When you have the feeling that something is lying on the surface of your arms, and that it flies up into the air when you make the movement for *c*, then you have something which can lead you to a more or less true experience of the *c*-movement.

D, as I told you, is a pointing downwards, or indeed a pointing in any direction: *d*; if one now adds to this sound the sound *a*, so that wonder is aroused by that towards which one points, then one gets the word: *da*.

Now imagine for a moment that we wished to express the nature of the Oriental teacher. The Oriental teacher—particularly the older Oriental teacher—is indeed quite different from the European teacher. To-day, in the case of the European, one always has the feeling that his whole educational system is based on the idea of pumping his pupils, of drawing all manner of things out of them. He meddles with them. To-day people talk about the necessity of ' developing ' the pupil, although this is idle talk for the most part. When one hears these modern educators expounding their pedagogic theories, one gets the feeling that one is, to use an Austrian expression, a *Zwirnskäuerl* (a ball of thread), and that one is being unwound. Indeed, when education is spoken of to-day one feels as if one were being absolutely torn to pieces. One is driven, crammed,— in short, there is no end to what is being done to those who are being educated. The European educator feels that he must make the human being into something utterly different from what he really is. If it were possible to carry out all that one hears talked about on all sides by those interested in the art of education, then the human being who finally emerged from their hand would indeed be a strange being! The attitude of the Oriental towards the teacher is different. He feels that the teacher, the educator, is one who points things out to his pupils, who draws their attention to things and says: ' *Das ist das* ' (That is that). The Oriental teacher leaves his pupils unmolested because he assumes that they develop out of their own being and may, therefore, safely be let alone. Things are only pointed out to them. For this reason the Oriental teacher is one who, whatever he is doing, always says, as it were, ' da '; *da-da*—der Dada. And this is what he is called. The oriental teacher is called the ' Dada '. It is his mission to point everything out: *da-da!*

Now looking at modern civilization,—which, from a certain point of view, is progressing in a way that I can only describe as inverse to Darwinism,—we see that humanity, having satisfactorily arrived at the theory of man's descent from the ape, desires to return to the ape once more, thus progressing quite clearly in a contrary direction to Darwinism. The tendency is to return once again to the primitive, to the primeval. In consequence there has arisen a sort of ' Dada-ism '. Some years ago, when I was in Berlin, I received a letter in which the writer signed himself ' Der Ober-Dada ' (the Head Dada). This is a retrogression, a principle of imitation, such as is found in this inverse Darwinism, this returning once more to the ape. You see how it is; one just imitates. And so, in founding this sort of ' Dada-ism ' in Europe one is really imitating the more primitive methods of the Oriental.

In the word ' dada ', however, there does actually lie some expression of this educating gesture, of this drawing attention to something, pointing to something. (Frl. S. . . . will you show us the movement for *d*? Try to enter right into the nature of the *d*-sound). What is really the nature of the *d*-sound? In it there lies the indicating movement. Thus you must have the feeling: *There* is something; *there* is something else; *d*,—when you finally land on it.—For this reason you must carry out the movement in such a way that there is a certain harmony between the two arms. One arm must reach a definite point just a moment before the other. The arm that starts later, however, must follow on quickly as though being drawn by the arm which started earlier. The direction of the movement may be either towards the left or towards the right.

It is very necessary to study these things in detail, and you must learn really to *feel* this indicating, this pointing towards

68

something. But first, in order to express the *d*-sound successfully, you must accustom yourselves to this pointing; you must introduce this pointing. The hands must be held in this way (pointing with the finger.)

I told you yesterday that *f* is really Isis. In *f* there is the consciousness of being permeated with wisdom. When one first feels one's own inner being and then experiences this inner being in the process of out-breathing, in the outgoing breath stream,—*f*,—then one has the true *f*. Man experiences the wisdom of his own being, that is to say, of his own etheric body, in the out-breathing process. This feeling must be present in the movement which represents the *f*-sound. (Frau P . . . . will you make an *f*.) This movement corresponds exactly to the movement which the utterance of the *f*-sound produces in the air as it is breathed outwards. You must make the movement for *f* in such a way that there is a break in it; then only will you feel what I have indicated with regard to the nature of *f*. You must show that there is, as it were, a second attack in the sound. But do not make the movement so quickly; it must be gentler. That is the *f*. In the movement for *f* we have a very exact imitation of this conscious out-breathing process which is of such great significance.

Now I have already told you that in the *l* we have the sound which actually forms something, the sound in which we feel the form-giving process with the tongue. *l-l-l*. In order to make this clear I took the word *leim* (glue) as an example; I pointed out the adhesive quality of this substance, its formative quality, the capacity it has for imitating form, in other words, the way in which it strives to represent the fundamental nature of the *l*-sound. *L* was looked upon in the Mysteries as a sound possessing special magical qualities, for when one gives form to something it follows that one has power over it. And it was just this aspect of *l*, this quality of mastering something, of gaining power over something which, in the Mysteries, caused this sound to be looked upon as one containing demonic forces. All this must be embodied in the movement for *l*. And when, added to this, you feel as if your arms are quite supple, flexible in themselves; when you feel that something takes place in the arms which is similar to the movement of your tongue when you say *l*,— then you will experience *l* in the right way, and you will discover that there is something truly fascinating in this movement.

Then we have the sound *m*. I said yesterday that *m* signifies the understanding of something, the capacity for entering into something with intelligence. I told you that in the place where I was brought up it was customary to say *mhn; hn*, when one had heard something said and wished to emphasize the fact that one had understood it. *Mhn; hn*— we will discuss this further; it expresses the feeling of joy and satisfaction aroused by having understood something. And one really has the feeling of being absolutely devoured by the intelligence and understanding of the person to whom one is speaking when he says *mhn*. Hence, in the *m* of the sacred Indian word *Aum*, *m*, we have a marvellous expression of the understanding of the universe. Thus *m* may be said to signify the grasp of a thing: first there is the feeling of grasping something, then there is the penetration into it and lastly there follows the understanding of it. The position should be held for a moment, so that this intelligent comprehension which comes about as a matter of course is shown by the movement. (The arms should be held slightly in front of the body.)

It would indeed be wonderful if this movement could also be taught to the elephant. The elephant could make a wonderful *m* by stretching its trunk outwards and then turning it under. One could not have a more perfect example of an *m*. An *m* carried out in this way would really be the best *m* one could possibly imagine. I mention all these things as they may help you really to experience the sounds.

The uneasy sort of feeling which one has when meeting a person with a nose like an eagle's beak will not be unknown to you. You will realize that a nose of this type really is the unconscious expression of the *m*-movement. The nose takes on the form of *m*. People with such a nose often cause a certain embarrassment to their fellows, because they give the impression of an absolute understanding of those with whom they come in contact, and it is not always pleasant to feel that one is being so completely understood. We get this feeling with people having an eagle-like nose for the simple reason that such a nose is really the *m*-movement held fast and frozen into a set form. He, however, who experiences the *m*-gesture in comprehending, even if this meets us in the form of an eagle-like nose, even if the eurythmy of the *m* already meets us in his nose,—this will not shatter us; rather one feels embarrassed.

But there is another kind of understanding, an understanding mingled with a feeling of repulsion, an understanding tinged with irony. Here one comprehends the matter in question, at the same time, however, revealing this attitude of mind: Why make such a fuss about it? Of course, it is absolutely obvious!—*n*. If you should happen to be in Berlin you could not fail to notice this. The impression that one has in Berlin is that people are not altogether pleased with one's affairs, but that they understand them perfectly! They immediately put everything on one side: *ne*. Indeed, the people of Berlin, if they know you well, say precious little besides *ne!* They really have not much else to say. This expression gives some indication of the attitude of mind of those who have a tendency to despise anything and everything which they feel they can understand as a matter of course.

One feels at once, when seeing this movement: The thing is of no importance. I understand it perfectly. And the eurythmist also must have this feeling. In order to get into the right mood for the *n*-movement, you should imagine that you are dealing with someone who is quite stupid, someone who in his conversation keeps laying great emphasis upon the most ordinary things. You want to make him realize that he really is too stupid, that you can understand the matter very quickly and wish to get away from the whole thing as soon as possible. That is the experience.

I have already told you that *r* is the sound which expresses the complete turning over of something; it is the expression

71

of something which is not itself round, but which takes on a rounded form. One always has the feeling that this is difficult to imitate, because the most natural way to make the movement for *r* would be to turn a complete somersault, and this, of course, we cannot do! Frl. S. . . . will you show us the movement for *r*? That is a very strenuous *r*. It is one way of doing it. Now Frl. S. . . . will you show us another *r*? That is another way of doing it. So you see there are various ways of expressing the movement very beautifully; it is a turning, revolving movement, which takes place in the breath-process also, for there is indeed a rolling movement when the sound *r* is uttered.

Such, then, are the things which I believe may show you to some extent, and in an introductory way, how through eurythmy the gestures of ordinary experience can be led over into formed movements, into movements which really have form and shape.

LECTURE 4

THE INDIVIDUAL SOUNDS AND THEIR COMBINATION INTO
WORDS

Dornach, 27th June 1924

I think that in yesterday's lecture we reached the point at
which we were considering the sound *r*, and I had previously
unfolded before you the inner nature of most of the other
sounds.

It is important above all that we should learn to understand the *s*-sound. *S* as we learned yesterday, was always
looked upon in the Mysteries as a sound of the very highest
importance. Indeed, it was looked upon as possessing
magical qualities; for it can be felt as a sound which brings
with it surety and certainty, a feeling of calm, a quietening
element. This is induced by the fact that, with the impulse
lying behind the sound *s* one can penetrate into the inmost
nature of another being.

For this reason I said that when a pupil of the old Mysteries
was asked by someone from the outer world what he had
learned through the *s*-sound, he answered, as was customary
at that time, in a somewhat humorous vein, and said: He
who is master of the *s*-sound can see into the souls of men
and into the hearts of women. There can be no question
that in both cases this insight entails the necessity of bringing about a feeling of calm. And this led quite naturally to
the humorous use of a sentence such as the one I have
described.

Now if in the *f*-sound we have the feeling: Wisdom lives
in me, wisdom created me, I breathe out wisdom, wisdom is
ever present within me,—then behind the *s*-sound we may
say that there lies a slight element of fear, something against
which we feel we must be on our guard. This is why in those
scripts,—in which, as I have already told you the *s*, or the

73

snake-like curved line is to be found in the various letters—writing was felt to be something uncanny, something which threw light into hidden depths. And to-day—using this word ' to-day ' in the sense of an historical epoch—certain peoples still exist (though naturally very few) who, unaccustomed as they are to the art of writing, regard the written characters as being distinctly uncanny. When the Europeans, these ' superior people ' of civilization, went to the North American Indians, the North American Indians found much that to them was unpleasant in the ways of these ' superior people ', and the written characters were among those things which produced in them such an unpleasant sensation. They made it quite clear that in their opinion these ' Pale Faces ', as they called them, these strange, foreign ' Pale Faces ' conjured ' little demons ' on to the paper. And as late as the nineteenth century there were certain Indian tribes who still regarded the printed letters as being the embodiment of little demons.

Let us consider these two sounds, these two letters, the f and the s. They must be formed in eurythmy in such a way that the onlooker can perceive a tremendous difference between them. When the movement for f is made, it must express the quiet sense of power over that which has been conjured up in the world by its means. The movement is created out of an element of peace. The hands must bend over a little towards the arm, but in an active manner.

They must not hang passively, but must be held as if covering something and protecting it.

Now s. You see in the s-sound how something is, as it were, moved out of its course with a sense of mastery. (The movement was demonstrated.) The cause for this feeling really lies in the relationship which arises between the two arms as a result of the movement.

Now let us pass on to sch. One could hardly fail to recognize the blowing past, the blowing away of something, as this is expressed in the sound sch. I made this quite clear to you when I gave as an example the feeling lying behind

74

the word *husch-husch:* the breeze wafts by and passes away: *husch-husch*.

But everywhere in words of an interjectional character you will observe how this *sch* sound conveys this feeling of blowing past. There are indeed many words which in this connection are extraordinarily characteristic.

You must now consider the deep significance of something which I have already spoken about during these days, I mean the fact that in different languages things are called by different names. The reason for this is that the different languages are really describing different things. For instance, when in German I say the word *kopf*, this indicates the form, the plastic form of the head; when, on the other hand the word *testa* is used in Italian it signifies what takes place by means of the head, it signifies a process of corroboration, of affirmation. Thus the two languages are describing completely different things. That which is called *kopf* in German would also be called *kopf* in Italian, if the Italian wished to express the same idea.

In this way languages differ very much from each other. When we take the German language we find that it is of a plastic nature. The genius of the German language is really a sculptor. This must not be overlooked. The peculiar characteristic of the German language is that it is plastic: the genius of the language is a sculptor.

The genius of the Latin languages has, on the other hand, something of the lawyer about it, something of the advocate, of one who affirms, confirms, testifies.

This is in no way intended as a criticism, but merely as a description of certain characteristics. Each language contains within it the temperament and character of its genius. One may actually carry this so far as to say that when one hears Hungarian, Magyar or Finnish spoken, one cannot fail to have the feeling that something is really lacking. It is impossible to listen to the Magyar language without feeling that after every third word something is lacking. When the Hungarian or Magyar language is spoken one feels that after every third word a stag should be shot. The reason for this is that the genius of the Hungarian language is a hunter. In the Magyar language all words which have not arisen out of the activity of the hunt are in reality borrowed. The Magyar language has absorbed many such words, and when one arrives in Budapest one finds at once among the names written up in the streets such strange words as, for example: *Kaveház*. (From the German: *Kaffeehaus*: Café). Such words as these have not, of course, the characteristic I have described; the Magyar language has adopted many such borrowed words. But when one listens to the Magyar language, it is certainly imbued with the element of the hunt, of the chase. Naturally there is nothing bad about this; the tiller of the soil, the hunter and the shepherd are invariably the source from which the whole human race has arisen. There still lives a primeval force in such a language as that of the Magyars. And the genius of the Magyar language is undoubtedly a hunter, or, if you will, a huntress, Diana.

So we can say, in the German language we have the plastic formative element; that is a feature which is very much in evidence. For this reason we find many interjections, which are uncommonly characteristic. Well, it does not even need to be a snake,—even if a restless, agitated mouse is hidden under some leaves, we have already something moving and rolling about, and it gives us an uneasy sensation, we are astonished: *r-a*—now it scampers away: *sch*. The feeling of astonishment is not all, however; something is done to us, but we bear up under it: *e*. Now whatever is moving in this way clings to its surroundings, it adapts itself to them, burrows its way through; where there is a hollow space it makes its way through, creeping now lower, now higher: *l*. And when it emerges, then we understand what it was all about: *n. rascheln* (to rustle). Here you have the whole story of *rascheln* in plastic form.

The remarkable feature of the German language is that one can find in it so much that really corresponds to plastic art, that really makes up the plastic element of language. Hence it is perhaps not without significance that eurythmy, in the first instance, could most easily arise within the German language, for eurythmy may be said to be sculpture brought into the realm of movement, and it is from out of the German language that this living sculpture can be most easily developed at the present day. In ancient times all languages possessed a living, plastic element. It is true that other languages are more musical in their nature, as is the case, for instance, with the Magyar language. The German language cannot be said to be musical, but for this very reason the plastic element is all the stronger.

And it is just in this word *rascheln*, as also in the ' husch-husch ', that we have the blowing away, the blowing past, the scattering of something.

The Hebrew man of ancient times experienced in the *sch* the presence of Jehovah in the blowing of the wind: *sch*. Naturally this also may be felt as lying behind the plastic eurythmic movement for the sound *sch*. The movement must be rapid, then it has the true ' rustling ' effect, (*rascheln*), and really gives the feeling that is expressed in the word. It is no exaggeration to say that one actually hears the rustling in the form of the movement.

Yesterday I spoke to you also about the way in which the sound *z* is to be understood. I said then that there is a certain lightness in the experience of *z*. And this experience, together with its plastic, eurythmic expression, is derived from this feeling of lightness, from something which is essentially light. Thus, when we turn our attention to *z* we shall regard it in much the same way as one might do a child, who, having lost a new toy which has been bought for it, cries and is inconsolable. One would not wish to scold the child, but to comfort it. Let us suppose that it is not the mother or the father who is dealing with the child, but an aunt or grandmother, whose manner towards the child (who has been up to some mischief) is aunt-like, or grandmotherly. The gesture, especially with the right hand, suggests: Never mind, little one. . . . It would be quite good if we were to bear such little stories in mind. You must feel the *z* more especially in the arm; not in the wrist, but in the downward movement of the arm.

Up to now, my dear friends, we have mainly considered the nature of the individual sounds as such. At this point it will be necessary for us to discover the right way of expressing the *connection between* the sounds; and in order to lead over gradually into this somewhat different sphere, I shall from time to time take the opportunity of making certain observations. As occasion offers I shall deviate from the purely artistic side of eurythmy and refer to educational, and also to curative eurythmy. Thus, when I pass over to educational eurythmy, you will see how this aspect of eurythmy must be derived from the inner nature of the sounds as we have studied them in these lectures. It is quite obvious that in the beginning, when teaching the movements, one should as far as possible choose words expressing a definite mood or feeling. So that one enters into the spirit of eurythmy by means of the *feeling contained in the sounds*, and by this means we are able to conjure up a right attitude towards eurythmy, a realization that eurythmy is a language, a language which may indeed be understood if only approached without prejudice. Now everything is contained for us in this word *rascheln*, if you make the movement as clearly as possible, and with great precision; only you must never lose sight of the fact that it is not the external process only which is of importance, but that the movements must be permeated by feeling. When this word is shown now in eurythmy I shall be able to tell you what is really contained within it just at one particular point,—and then you will indeed perceive what is hidden in this word. . . . ! (The word was demonstrated.) Now, for instance, the person who has been disturbed by the rustling pokes his nose in the direction from which it comes!

So you see, when we take into account the subjective element of feeling, we find that absolutely everything is contained in eurythmy.

We will now take another very characteristic word. You will remember my description of the sound *c* (ts); *k* is similar, but stronger. In the sound *k*, we have matter governed, mastered, by spirit. Suppose for a moment that you are confronted by a regular termagant, by somebody who appears all physical strength and of whom you are somewhat afraid. It is not easy to deal with such a person; but, although you have to brace yourself against his behaviour, you, nevertheless, wish to get rid of him,—to, as it were, ' blow him away '. You say to him then, but in eurythmy, *kusch*. In this word you have every possibility of feeling these things; there is the repulsing of the person in question, the feeling of gathering one's self together in order to confront him, but there is also the mastery over him. In practising the word do it in such a way that you have a very clear *sch* at the end. For the pacifying element in the word *kusch* lies in the fact that one intends to get rid of something.

Now, in teaching eurythmy, it is important to choose those words in which one can on the one side still feel the plastic formation of the sounds, and on the other side the inner life that is thereby developed.

Now these sounds make up in themselves the separate elementary parts of eurythmy as a whole. From these parts words are then put together. When, in a word, let us say, for instance, the word *rascheln*, you simply make the sounds in an intellectual manner one after another, the result will not be a word in the true sense. It is an undeniable fact that a word is much more of a complete whole than one usually thinks. If this were not so, we, as speaking human beings, could never have become so dried up and lifeless as we unfortunately are. When we read aloud, we do not read the individual sounds quite distinctly; we glide over the whole word and only touch lightly upon the single sounds. The one sound passes over into the other; and in ordinary speech also, the one sound passes over into the next. In eurythmy, therefore, we must not only pay particular attention to the forming of the single sounds, but above all, to the movement which expresses the transition from sound to sound. A word can only become beautiful in eurythmy if one succeeds in obtaining a natural transition from one sound to the next.

And so it becomes necessary to turn our attention to the way in which one sound proceeds out of the other. One should try to discover how this takes place, and for this reason it is good to take characteristic words, which occur very often, practising them, not so much from the point of view of the individual sounds, but as a whole.

Take, for instance, the word *und* (and), the simple word *und* and try to show it in one continuous, unbroken movement. Try, before you have quite finished the *u*-sound, to begin the *n*. This lends itself very well to eurythmy. Before the movement for *u* is really completed, let it pass over into *n*: *u-n*,—and from this immediately make the transition into the *d*: *und*.

From a study of eurythmy it is really possible to discover the inner intentions of the genius of language. I told you that *d* is the indicating movement. This is shown clearly in eurythmy. Now how does the word *und* end? It ends with *d*, with the indicating movement. What purpose does the word *und* really serve? We say, for instance, ' sun and moon '. There is the sun. We turn from the sun to the moon, indicating the moon by means of the ' and '. Thus through eurythmy one is able to re-discover the primeval gestures underlying speech. All this must be felt and experienced.

Bearing this in mind, let us take a word that even in the German language has long lost its plastic form, which, however, it once possessed to a very high degree. When I say ' once ', that does not mean centuries ago; I refer to a not so very distant past. At that time this word had a plastic form. It is true that the word as we now know it is comparatively modern, but as it emerged from the dialect it still had its plastic character. And as dialect it still retains this character to-day. As I said before we must not allow our feeling for such things to be disturbed by a philology which in its own place is fully justified. Let us take this German word *Mensch* (human being), and let us express it in eurythmy, somewhat shortening the final *sch*-sound: *Mensch*. Here we have a distinct feeling of the blowing past at the end of the word.

How do the eurythmy movements for this word affect us?

They give us the impression of the transience of human life; they give us a picture of the fleeting nature of man. Carrying this somewhat farther, we are shown the insignificance of the human being; this is what the eurythmic gestures say to us when showing the word *Mensch* as a whole.

Now in dialect the word *Mensch* signifies a woman of completely trivial character. The word is not used in any bad sense, but simply indicates a woman who is quite uninteresting: *das Mensch*. Here the element of insignificance is strongly emphasized, and the tragic conception which one has regarding *der Mensch* is carried further and coloured with contempt when one says: *das Mensch*.

Thus in the plastic gestures and movements of eurythmy we have the possibility of learning to feel deeply the meaning and true nature of words.

There is one thing, however, about which we must be perfectly clear. Eurythmy, by means of the sounds which make up the different words, necessarily leads us into the inner nature of that to which the sounds themselves refer. When you see words for apparently the same thing shown in eurythmy, you will nevertheless perceive, by the character of the movements, the difference in the character of the words. Will Frl. B. . . . and Frl. W. . . . now stand side by side, and we will ask Frl. B. . . . first to show the word *kopf*, and afterwards Frl. W. . . . will show *testa*. Now with the word *kopf* you have the feeling that the eurythmist wishes to form something round, wishes to be a sculptor. The eurythmist who is showing the word *testa* is determined to be in the right! In this way you see visibly expressed the essential characteristics of any particular word.

These things must be borne in mind. Then you will discover how, through eurythmy, the character of the different languages is revealed in a most subtle and marvellous way. You can feel how the character of the different languages rises up, as it were, before your very eyes.

In order that this may be more fully illustrated, let us now see a German, an English, a French, and possibly also a

81

Hungarian and a Russian poem interpreted in eurythmy; in such a way, moreover, that by emphasizing as far as possible all the sounds, the character of the poem in question is clearly shown. (The poems were then demonstrated by representatives of the different nations.) You will at once perceive how, for instance, the English language reveals its connection with the waves of the sea. And the mastery of the waves, which lies so strongly in the English language, comes out extraordinarily clearly in eurythmy.

In the Magyar language, the feeling, the mood which is brought to expression is that the Magyar can only picture himself as being planted firmly on the earth, and having to roam through thicket and forest. This, too, you can see in the interpretation of the Magyar poem.

Russian, again, is a language which is merely suggestive, which only gives a faint indication of the inner nature of the word. It is a language which has not yet its true being, but is following the tracks leading it towards this being, and is pointing on all sides towards the future.

And now I should like you to compare two things which will give you an insight into the marked way in which this difference of character reveals itself. One must learn to feel this, otherwise one cannot find one's way into the nature of eurythmy. A purely theoretical, intellectual explanation will not suffice; we must be led to a true feeling and understanding of what eurythmy really is. Let us then compare the eurythmic interpretation of a Russian poem with that of a French poem. Try to realize the great contrast between the two. (The Russian poem was here demonstrated.) Now with the Russian poem you see how one *follows on the tracks* of the word, and try now with the other poem, the French poem, to observe how there is, as it were, even in front of a word, a *tripping away* from it. (The French poem was then demonstrated.) Here there is the feeling of always being in front of the word. You see these two languages may really be compared to day and night, to the opposite poles, their characteristics are so different.

When you consider all these things, which are really quite apparent, you will feel bound to say: In eurythmy there is the possibility of bringing clearly to expression the living spirit which is embodied in language, and above all the *character* of the language. For this reason eurythmy is particularly well fitted to express all that lies *behind* language. And one must, of course, be able to express what lies behind language.

In this connection we will take our start from something quite definite. We differentiate, when we speak in this way, between abstract words, words which indicate the abstract, and words which indicate the concrete. The point is that with words indicating something abstract the play of feeling is quite different from concrete words. If one has an unprejudiced, lively perception, if one is neither a frog nor a fish—and without being either frog or fish listens to speech—then one has, in the case of an abstraction, the feeling of being hollowed out, of becoming empty. One becomes inwardly glacial when one hears abstractions. Naturally one must cultivate a sensitiveness for this. One should, for example, even develop sensitiveness for things which, when uttered, must be said to sound paradoxical. But whoever will live into language, and thereby into eurythmy, in an artistic way, he must be able to form just such sensitive inner perceptions.

People read Kant—now you are all educated people and you know, do you not, even if you have not read Kant yourselves, what a figure one must make of oneself if one reads Kant (Mirth, Heiterkeit). Well, why does this strike you as so humorous? You think one can't do that. I will prove to you at once that one can do it, quite adequately. It is only so disagreeable to read Kant in the town or in a reading room or lecture room. He does not fit in here. But try just once, when it is really cold, to read Kant on Mont Blanc: then you will see at once how adequate this is. Isn't it so, when you begin Kant it is abstract, when you end Kant it is abstract. If you actually read him in the icy atmosphere, there he fits in admirably, he fits in there,—if you can think of such a thing,—there the feeling is out and out suited to the abstract.

The concrete must not be read on Mont Blanc, but this must be read or spoken by the warm stove. This does not hollow one out but one is replenished.

Background

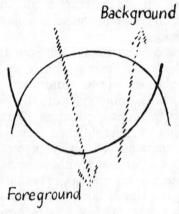

Foreground

And now just try, in a connection in which something must be conceived as abstract, really to indicate the abstraction. Let us first show an abstract word. Naturally all this is relative, for what is abstract for one person can be very concrete for another. But now let us take something very abstract, and you indicate for us the gestures, the movement, that is to say, for the abstraction in general. We will suppose, for example, that in some connection there appeared the word "triangle" and you wanted to show its abstraction. You must do this in such a way (see diagram) that, if this is background and this foreground (see diagram), this movement would appear (the movement was stepped in space). You take on yourself the unpleasant task of hollowing something out; you build, as it were,—if I express myself in a drastic manner, the front part of a barrel—so that you have not got the wine in front of you, but behind you, so that you cover it. The front part of a barrel makes the abstraction.

Now make the concrete, let us say, for example ' frog '

or ' fish ,' anything we like,—for everything is concrete that can be seen. Now the essential nature of the concrete is this movement (see diagram). When you do this movement then you can give the impression that you have the wine in front of you. You take it into your care. You feel in yourself that which represents replenishment.

Suppose we wished to show in eurythmy a strong feeling of affirmation.

A young man leaves his parents' house. They declare, as he bids them farewell, that he will come back again: You will come back to us again,—says the father. Try now to express in eurythmy this phrase: You will come back to me again,—and in doing so show clearly the feeling of affirmation. How do we express this? By a step. When we wish to affirm something we take a step *forwards* (towards the right) and in this step there must be the feeling, as it were, of the *i*-sound, of assertion. Thus affirmation is expressed by a movement of the foot from the back forwards.

Negation,—let us suppose that somebody tells a child he is not to do something: You must never do that again . . . . If you wish to emphasize this feeling of negation, you must do so by taking a step backwards (towards the left). These things are, of course, quite elementary.

Thus we can pass over from what is revealed as to the nature of the single word to the inner logic which is contained in language. And in this way the character of the language becomes still more evident. If one considers the single sound as such, when expressing a poem in eurythmy in any language, then the character of the *language* is emphasized.

When, on the other hand, we take into consideration things which we shall be studying presently, when we pass over to logic as it is expressed in language, then more emphasis is laid on the character of the *people*.

Let us pass over now to this logic of language, and to begin with take the feeling of wonder. When a passage occurs in which the feeling of wonder is expressed, you will make the movement for wonder (movement for *a*) and you must merge the movement in with the other sounds, so that both mood and sounds are shown. Much study is required before one succeeds in expressing the succession of sounds, together with the indication of the logic of language, of the emotional content.—*Ach wie schön* (O how beautiful)!—Try here to put the two things together, the movement for wonder and the sounds contained in the words: '*Ach, wie schön!*'*—

The movement expressing wonder must be united with the actual single sounds; wonder must lie in the formation of the sound.

To-morrow we will analyse other similar movements.

* According to feeling and mood other vowels might of course also be chosen to add colour to the whole; these would likewise have to be blended in with the actual succession of sound.

Dornach, 30th June 1924

To-day we will continue our study of those things with which we have already made a beginning in the previous lecture. We took as our starting point the inner feeling and mood of the individual sounds, and from this we passed over to the more general characteristics of speech. In so doing we considered not only the sounds as such, but also the feeling lying behind them, or their logical content.

In this lecture I shall not be dealing so much with the single sounds, but I shall speak about the mood and feeling which may be called up within us by a poem taken as a whole. In the first place—later we shall gather the different threads together,—in the first place, we have something which can serve to bring out the finer nuances and shades of feeling which arise out of the word, out of the way in which the different sounds are put together. We can, for instance, say something aloud, and, by emphasizing one word more than another, show by our manner of speaking the feeling lying behind the actual words. It is obvious that much depends upon emphasis, and in writing, this emphasis is shown by such things as question marks, exclamation marks, and so on.

The simple little example which follows will give you an insight into the importance of correct emphasis. If I remember rightly, in Szegedin, in Hungary, there was once a company of actors who were giving a performance of Schiller's *Räuber*, in a barn, of all places, next door to a cattle shed. One of the actors did not know the text perfectly, and was also unable to understand the prompter. The prompter's text may have been inaccurate; in any case, the whole affair was somewhat primitive. And the amateurish effect was not lessened when a regular dispute took place in the presence of the audience. This dispute arose owing to the fact that one of the oxen suddenly broke through the wall and gazed around, so that its horns and muzzle were visible on the stage. At this moment the actor, who was somewhat alarmed, said, looking in the direction of the cow: ' *Seid Ihr auch wohl mein* Vater? ' (Are you indeed my *father?*) The prompter corrected him, saying: Should he not say: *Seid Ihr auch* wohl, *mein Vater?*) (Are you *well*, my father?) And that did not please the stage manager, who made the following correction: Here he should say: ' Seid *Ihr auch wohl mein Vater?* (*Can* you be my father?)

So you see everything depends upon emphasis. And as we must be able to express in eurythmy all the fundamental elements of language, it must also be possible to express what in speech would be brought about by means of emphasis, and in writing by means of the question mark, the exclamation mark, or something of that kind. To fulfil this need we have a movement which gives rise to a feeling similar to that called up in written language by the exclamation or the question mark. This movement must be carried out in the following way.

The eurythmist places both the right and left arm in the position indicated in the diagram, the left hand being turned slightly inwards and the fingers held loosely. (see p. 90).

This then is a movement which should be made use of as occasion offers. I shall speak about colour in eurythmy later on. Now, of course, the eurythmist must only make use of this movement at suitable moments, and the way in which it is used must be very carefully studied. For instance, the eurythmist must come to an understanding with the reciter, so that a slight pause is made in the reading. And it must be done in such a way that the onlooker can see clearly that the eurythmist is here passing over from the movement, first into a relative, and then into a complete state of rest; so that the movement brings about a distinct break in the poem. For example, if I say: ' How lovely the sunshine is to-day! We must make the most of it.'—the point would be to express the exclamation adequately. Therefore, at the point where the exclamation mark is, you would bring the movement, which otherwise is in constant flow, to a standstill. You would take up this position quite quietly, and then proceed. Such an example offers a good opportunity for the clear expression of this movement.

An excellent opportunity for applying this movement is to be found in such a poem as Goethe's *Zauberlehrling*, where many exclamations occur. In this poem the movement would serve to bring out what may be called humour in the truly artistic sense of that word. For instance, at the end of the line: ' *In die Ecke, Besen, Besen, seid's gewesen!*'—the movement for the exclamation is strongly called for; and again at the end of the next line: ' *Denn als Geister. . . .!* ' When the magician himself is speaking, the movement would not be suitable, for he is a stately personage. But it would be particularly good if the eurythmist who is interpreting the part of the pupil would introduce this movement quite frequently. Again it could be made use of after: ' *brav getroffen* ', and also after: ' *und ich atme frei!* '

There is another gesture expressing mood, which we may use when we wish to show *Liveliness* or *Mirth*. (Heiterkeit). You must carry out this gesture in such a way that you try, when making it, to stand on tip-toe. Thus, when the mirth is at its height, you must rise on the toes; and then, supposing this to be your head (See diagram) proceed to take up this position with your arms, spreading out your fingers. In this way we get the movement for *Mirth* or *Liveliness*.

When in addition to spreading out your fingers you move them about, the feeling of gaiety will be particularly well expressed. Such a movement gives the effect of merry laughter and possesses very great charm.

Let us take the following sentence: ' He went up into the reading desk, but before he could begin his lecture a fly settled on his nose! General consternation! ' (The movement should be made after the word ' nose '.) You see, even you who are behind the scenes and know all about it— (addressing one of the eurythmists present)—have succumbed to a very natural expression of mirth. And this

89

feeling of mirth, as it seems to me, is expressed remarkably
well by this movement.

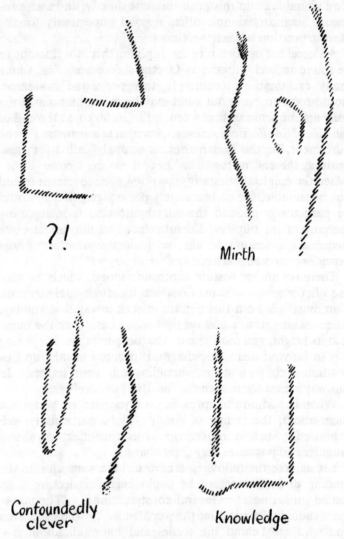

?!

Mirth

Confoundedly
clever

Knowledge

There are many opportunities in dialogue, in poems of a
dramatic nature, where you wish to make a dramatic effect,

when you can use another movement which is extraordinarily expressive. Picture the upper arm drawn downwards, with the forefinger pointing upwards, while the left arm is held pressed against the side. Picture this movement to yourselves. And now imagine that somebody says: ' I could have done that much more cleverly than you '—This could be expressed in eurythmy by the movement for ' *confoundedly clever* ' (Verflucht gescheit). This movement must be shown by making a sharp angle with the left arm, and pointing upwards with the right.

In these eurythmy figures you see before you the movements for the *Question* or *Exclamation*, *Mirth* and ' *confoundedly clever* '.*

Here (indicating the next figure), you have a movement which requires the closest study. The movement consists in bringing the hand and lower arm into this position (see diagram), with the first finger pointing upwards; for the characteristic feature of this movement is that it always indicates insight, discernment.

Whenever this movement makes its appearance it expresses insight; the finger, however, must not actually *point*, but it must be held in an upright position. In this way something of the movement for Cleverness is contained in this solemn gesture expressing *Knowledge*. (*Erkenntnis*).

When, therefore, you hold the right arm in an upright position, in the way I have described, and when you separate the rhythmic system and the head, which are chiefly concerned here, from the lower part of the human being, by holding the left arm across the body with the hand turned upwards as if to support the right elbow, then you have the complete movement for *Knowledge*. There are many opportunities for making use of this movement, for every word which indicates that one has perceived something, that one has absorbed something into one's being, can certainly be regarded as coming into the sphere of knowledge. The mood of a poem can be greatly enhanced when at the end of a line this gesture is used to show that the content of the poem

* The eurythmy figures carved in wood were shown in this connection.

has been absorbed and understood.   Many poems,—as for
example Uhland's *Des Sangers Fluch:*
    ' *Es stand in alten Zeiten ein Schloss so hoch und hehr . . . .* '
can gain very much if the eurythmist makes this movement
for Knowledge before actually beginning the text.   How
much has been added to the interest of a poem by introducing
such a movement at the beginning, will become apparent as
the poem proceeds.   Do it in such a way that your whole
body expresses the gesture for Knowledge.   From any
natural, simple position pass over into the gesture for
Knowledge.   By so doing, you develop the poem out of a
mood which in itself at once gives the key-note to the poem,
showing that its character is reflective and thoughtful.

There is another gesture of mood which rightly claims our
attention, one which lays special stress on the mood otherwise shown by the gesture for *i*—that is to say, the mood of
self-assertion.   *I* is always the assertion of self.   But when
the self-assertion does not lie in the *sound*, when it goes
beyond the sound into the general mood and feeling of the
poem, then it can be expressed in another way, by another
gesture.   In this gesture one must stand on the left leg, with
the right knee bent.   Both arms must be held in front of the
body, but in such a way that they are bent somewhat backwards, especially the hands.   Here we have the movement
expressing *exaggerated self-assertion.* (*Starke Selbstbe-
hauptung*).

Frl. V. . . . will you show the following sentence in eurythmy, passing at the end into this gesture, the gesture expressing the *wildest delusion*: 'Am I not the Emperor of China.
. . . ? ' Now for the movement!   This is how life can be
brought into what we have to express; and the essential,
the all-important thing is that eurythmy should be filled
with life.

I wanted to-day to bring before you such expressive gestures as these, so that we shall be able in the following
lectures to lead on without a break into a consideration of
much that is of the greatest interest.

There is yet another gesture which consists, in the first

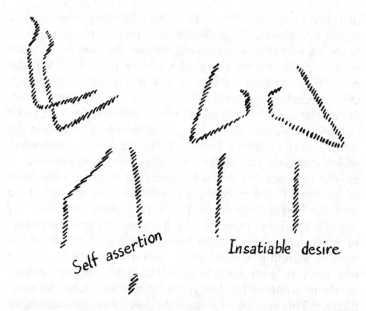

Self assertion   Insatiable desire

place, of making oneself appear as broad as possible. Then
one proceeds to make the movement for *Insatiable Desire*
(*Unersättlichkeit*) (see diagram), a movement which indicates
that one cannot get enough of something,—in other words
the gesture for intense desire.

Let us take, for instance, the following sentence, and when
I have come to the end of it, pass over immediately, as you
did before, into this gesture of craving for more. Let us
now take this quite serious sentence, and follow it with the
gesture: 'Thou gavest me everything, everything that I
asked of thee.' But you must not turn your hands outwards,
for that would express more the feeling of rejection. You
want more; the movement showing the desire for more
must be turned inwards, and you must make yourself as
broad as possible, standing with both feet firmly on the
earth.

One need not only apply this movement when one's own
feeling of longing is unappeased, but also when something
occurs giving rise to the feeling of craving, of dissatisfaction,

of the longing for more. Take the following sentence as I repeat it, and here also make the movement at the conclusion, in such a way that no pause ensues, but that you simply pass over into this movement at the end of the text: ' *Soll das ganze Haus ersaufen?* ' ('Is the whole house to be swamped?') (Corresponding gesture). There is to be no end to it. Hence the feeling of a demand which can never be satisfied.*

Now we come to those things which lead us more into the inward part of man's being. Here we have a movement which expresses *inwardness* of feeling, which is intended to express that mood of soul which manifests itself as inwardness of feeling. This may be shown by standing on the ball of the foot, the heel slightly raised above the ground, but only very slightly, for if it is raised too high it does not give the feeling of inwardness. Thus with heels raised slightly above the ground, standing on the ball of the foot, we should take up this position with both arms. The arms should be held gently in front of the body, the thumb touching the fore-finger. This gesture expresses the feeling of *Inwardness*, of *Tenderness*. (*Innigkeit*).

If you imagined to yourselves that you were holding a baby, and that you wanted to enter into a certain relationship with the guardian angel of this baby, you would hold it in this way, and you would then have the movement for *Inwardness*. Let us take a particularly solemn sentence and make this gesture at its close. Try to express in eurythmy: ' Come unto me all ye that labour and are heavy laden . . . ' and now the gesture. This is purely lyrical. If now you wish to raise the whole thing out of the lyric mood and give a grander impression, you can pass over from the movement for *Inwardness* to that of the *Exclamation*. Thus: ' Come unto me all ye that labour and are heavy laden—' now make the movement for *Inwardness* followed by that of the *Exclamation*. If these movements are carried out in the tempo which one feels to be suitable a very powerful impression will be created.

Something which in its feeling is closely related to the

* See Goethe's poem " Der Zauberlehrling."

mood of *Inwardness*, but which at the same time is quite different is the feeling of *Lovableness* (*Liebenswürdigkeit*), *charm*. This feeling is also expressed by raising the heels slightly from the ground; but the arms, while retaining to some extent the former position, are moved, the left arm being raised upwards, and the right arm drawn downwards. This then is the gesture for expressing the quality of *Lovableness*.

You must, however, feel that this really *is* the gesture which expresses lovableness. Very much depends upon holding the arms quite lightly, and in giving the feeling of really going out beyond oneself. I need only remind you how charming children can be when one coaxes them, and says: 'Come and show me how big you are!'—Children are never more delightful than at such a moment.

If we wished to show the following sentence in eurythmy: 'I have to thank your smile for a happy moment' . . . then it would be very appropriate to finish with the movement for *Lovableness*.

At one time, when in Vienna, I knew a certain composer, who has since become very famous. He liked very much to be invited out, and the hostess always exerted herself to provide him with the most delectable fare. She brought this to quite an art. This composer had a particularly fine appreciation for such things, and as a rule he said when taking his departure: 'What a glorious symphony we have partaken of to-day!'—That was always the compliment he paid to his hostess. It was a stereotyped compliment enough, but—he was a great man! Let us take the sentence and at its end make use of the gesture expressing *Charm*, *Lovableness*. You see that it goes absolutely by itself, and this example shows you how it can be felt. But the composer who was responsible for this saying would hardly have been able to make the movement with the same ease as an eurythmist, for it was no other than Brahms.

Another gesture which brings us into relationship with the outer world, with other human beings, is the one which we can make use of when we wish to impart something, when we

95

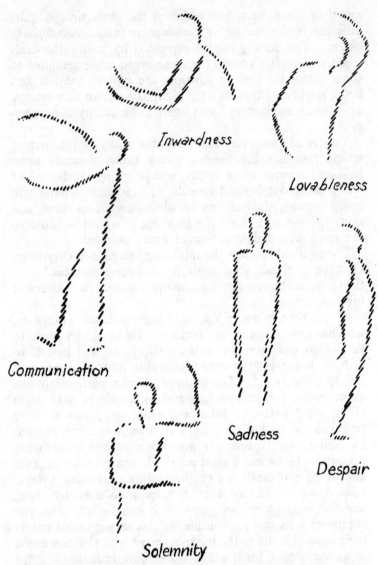

Inwardness

Lovableness

Communication

Sadness

Despair

Solemnity

wish to make a *Communication* (*Mitteilung*). This gesture is carried out in the following way. You must stand quite naturally on the one foot, the heel of the other foot, which is further forward, resting lightly on the ground. The right arm must be lifted up, with the thumb, first finger and middle finger pointing forwards; the left arm must be held lower, and must also be stretched somewhat outwards, towards the front, the palm of the hand turned upwards. This movement indicates that something is given; not an actual gift, but something is imparted by means of speech. There is, therefore, at the same time an indication of a gift, and here (in the left arm) the gesture of *Communication:* I communicate something.—This is the significance of the movement.

Let us take, for instance, the words: ' Verily, verily I say unto you '—Here we see very clearly the wish to impart something, to communicate something; and it is a wonderful opportunity for the use of this gesture of *Communication*.

Now we come to a movement, the character of which is shown when, at the appropriate moment, one stands firmly on the ground, the hands clenched, the arms stretched downwards and pressed against the body. The head should be held erect. In addition to this the eurythmist should try to have the feeling that the eyes are not actually looking at anything, that they are not actually seeing anything, but that the gaze is rigid and fixed. Then the movement will be very expressive. It is one which can often be made use of during the text of a poem:

> Blass lag der Kranke,
> Sein Auge erlosch,
> Schluchzen umgab ihn.

> (Pale was the sick man,
> Dim was his eye,
> Weeping friends surrounded him.)

The mood underlying such a sentence will be brought out particularly well if the eurythmist succeeds in making use of this movement in the places which I will here indicate with dots.

Blass lag . . . der Kranke,
Sein Auge . . . erlosch
Schluchzen . . . umgab ihn.

You will easily see how individual eurythmy can become when such movements are introduced, and how fine can be the nuances of its expression. This then is the movement for *Sadness* (Traurigkeit).

There is another movement which consists once more of standing firmly on both feet, with the arms held right back and the hands also right back. This is the movement for *Despair* (Verzweiflung); and you will very soon discover how strongly this feeling is expressed by the movement, particularly by the muscles of the inner arm. You will have the feeling: This is indeed the expression of despair.

Now we will try to do in eurythmy the first lines of the monologue in Faust, and after the word ' studiert ' we will make the movement for *Despair:*

Habe nun, ach! Philosophie,
Juristerei und Medizin
Und, leider! auch Theologie
Durchaus studiert.

I've studied now Philosophy
And Jurisprudence, Medicine,—
And even alas! Theology,—
From end to end, with labour keen.

Here make the movement for *Despair.* You see, when a movement really expresses the corresponding mood of soul, it indeniably enhances the dramatic effect of what has preceded it.

I should like to close to-day's lecture by saying a few words which may help to throw light on these movements and the way in which they should be studied. Study all such movements, then, by making use of them, you will be able to bring to plastic eurythmic expression many different shades of feeling. You will be able to enter more fully into the way in which a poem unfolds, and to study its dramatic, lyric or epic content. If you really feel your way into these movements, you will be able to bring a strong dramatic element into your eurythmy.

LECTURE 6

—The Inner Nature of Colour—

Dornach, 1st July 1924

Yesterday we concerned ourselves with various moods and shades of feeling and with the way in which these can be expressed by means of eurythmic gesture. To-day, to begin with, we will continue along somewhat similar lines. Taking our start from the point at which we left off yesterday, we will first consider the mood of *Devotion* or *Piety* (Andacht). It is very necessary, when trying to experience some such mood of soul, to realize that eurythmy does not attempt to interpret by means of ordinary mime. On the contrary, as we saw when studying the vowels and consonants, eurythmy seeks to draw the plastic form corresponding to such a feeling and mood from out of the whole human being, the whole human organization. We know that, in the case of the vowels and consonants, the movements are formed in such a way that they simply imitate and make visible what really exists as a kind of air form when the human being speaks. When we speak we make certain forms in the air. If by any means we were able to retain these forms and to hold them fast, we should have the original forms of the gestures which we use to express the sounds.

If, however, we wish to express some definite mood of soul, then we naturally approach much more closely to the arbitrary gesture, to the gesture which arises in ordinary, everyday life when we ourselves are experiencing the mood in question.

It is undeniable that to-day many people avoid the use of gesture, because, apparently, they have an idea that gesture is not the thing. On the other hand, however, the more the human being loses himself in feeling, the more he develops a mood of soul transcending the ordinary life of everyday, so much the more does the use of gesture become necessary. And such a mood of soul is that of *Devotion*.

In this devotional mood man has always felt the need for making a certain gesture. And the eurythmic gesture for *Devotion* is one which, in its very nature, corresponds to the instinctive attitude adopted when this mood arises in the soul. For this reason the eurythmic gesture for *Devotion* approximates more nearly to the naturalistic position than can be the case with most of the other movements. To express this mood of *Devotion* the arms are held downwards close to the body, and then bent upwards from the elbow, the hands and fingers taking up a position corresponding to one of the vowels, *u* for instance, or *a*. Thus according to the shade of feeling which one wishes to introduce into the mood of *Devotion*, any one of these postures may be adopted.

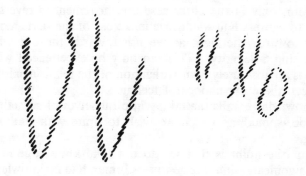

It is important that the gesture expressing this mood should be carried out in such a way that it is separated right off from the movements otherwise occurring in the course of the poem. So that in order to get the best effect it is as well in such a case to make use of the gesture at the beginning and again at the end of the poem. If, however, a devotional mood runs continuously through the whole of the prayer, the movement can be made at the beginning and at the end of every verse.

Will you now make use of this gesture when I say the following words:

> ' O Holy Spirit,
> Hearken to the cry of my soul! '

> Oh göttlicher Geist, erhöre
> meines Herzens Ruf!

The gesture should here be made both before and after the sentence. It would be especially good if the onlooker were actually to *see* how the upper arms are drawn downwards, pressed against the sides. This should precede the actual gesture for *Devotion*. (See diagram.)

An intensification of the mood of *Devotion* is the mood of *Solemnity*, of *Ceremonial* (Feierlichkeit). This mood of Solemnity is in a way not unlike the mood of Knowledge, of Wisdom, only in the latter case the movement is reversed. Thus to express Knowledge we make use of the same movement towards the right as we use towards the left when expressing Solemnity. This can only be experienced when there is an absolutely clear realization of the relation existing between these two moods of feeling.

Knowledge entails the taking into ourselves of something outside, something which we wish to unite with our own being.

Thus the point is that we do not take knowledge in its deep significance into the gesture. If man had no knowledge he could not be said to be man at all. It is through the capacity for absorbing knowledge that he first becomes truly human. So that knowledge, wisdom, should be looked upon as something which adds to the dignity of man, but which, on the other hand, contains within it a certain activity of soul. Activity is always expressed in eurythmy by turning towards the right. If we take the mood of

102

Knowledge and change it, making it more passive, more devotional, we get the feeling of *Solemnity*.

But wherever the passive element enters in, wherever there is little feeling of activity, then we turn towards the left and make our movements towards the left. And it is in this way that we express the mood of *Solemnity*. We make a movement similar to that of *Knowledge*, but in this case towards the left. Let us take an example in which we can make use of this gesture.

> ' Over the destiny of man
> Shine the inviolable stars. . . . '

> ' Über menschlichen Schicksalen
> Glänzen heil'ge Sterne '.

Here you should make the gesture both at the beginning and at the end. Begin by indicating the gesture for *Knowledge* and then carry it over into that of *Solemnity*.

In eurythmy we have chiefly to do with the expression and revelation of certain qualities of soul; and we shall see that the whole content of the soul life may be divided into three categories, into *Thinking*, *Feeling* and *Willing*. Now it is important, when interpreting a poem, really to express its fundamental character, and when this character changes in the course of a poem,—when, for example, thinking passes over into feeling, or feeling into will,—it is then very important that this should be shown in the whole bearing and in the character of the movements.

Let us take to begin with the two polar opposites, thinking and willing. They are indeed the most contrasted activities of the human soul. When the human being thinks,—I am speaking here in the widest sense of the word,—this is a process which depends upon the head as it rests quietly on the shoulders. By means of external sense-perception we cannot see the process of thought. It takes place in the quietly resting head. The activity of will is the extreme

103

opposite of this. When the activity of will does not make its appearance in the external world in some form or another, then it remains intention only. Real activity of will makes its appearance in the external world; such activity can be seen. But in so far as the inward experience of the human being is concerned, this will-activity remains dark, just as what takes place within the human being during the night remains dark to him. The human being knows nothing of his experiences as these take place during the night; he is just as little conscious of the relation between his soul and his muscles and bones, when some movement arises which is the expression of will-activity.

When you have a straight line you have something before you which is absolutely definite. You need only have a small portion of a straight line and its direction as a whole is absolutely determined. The straight line is something about which there can be no doubt whatever.

The curved line, on the other hand, is something which impels us to follow it, but we do not know exactly where it is going to lead us.

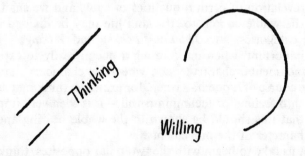

There are, it is true, regularly formed curved lines, but even in this case one experiences such regularity differently from the way in which one experiences the straight line. For this reason in eurythmy the straight line is used to denote thought and the curved line to denote will. You must, therefore, try to introduce straight lines into your form when you wish to express the element of thought and curved lines when you wish to express will-activity.

Now here, of course, much depends upon the eurythmist's conception of a poem. One might say: In this particular poem I intend to express the element of will. Another says, perhaps: I shall express thought, the imparting of something by means of thought. Two quite different conceptions! So in cases where the matter is not absolutely obvious the choice of interpretation lies in the hands of the individual eurythmist. This makes it necessary, when you begin to work out a poem, to put to yourselves the following question: What, in my opinion, is the fundamental character of this poem? Does it lean more towards thought? Does it impart something? Let us take, for example, the following:

Zu Aachen in seiner Kaiserpracht,
Im altertümlichen Saale,
Sass König Rudolfs heilige Macht
Beim festlichen Krönungsmahle.
Die Speisen trug der Pfalzgraf des Rheins,
Es schenkte der Böhme des perlenden Weins,
Und alle die Wähler, die sieben,
Wie der Sterne Chor um die Sonne sich stellt,
Umstanden geschäftig den Herrscher der Welt,
Die Würde des Amtes zu üben.

In this poem there is a succession of thoughts, as is usually the case with the pure epic. But if, at any point, the thought element were to pass over into the element of will, we should have to show this also in the eurythmic form. The particular verse I have just quoted, however, would best be expressed by moving as far as possible in straight lines.

Now it is, of course, also possible to combine straight lines in such a way that various figures are formed, so that you can introduce other characteristics beside thought by moving in a triangle, a square, or a pentagram as the case may be.

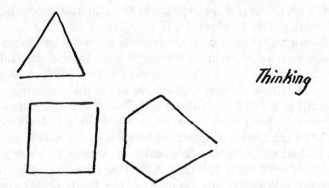

Thinking

On the other hand, if the thought is of a more complicated nature, you might perhaps make use of such a form as this:

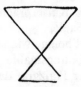

Every conceivable curved line serves to express the element of will.

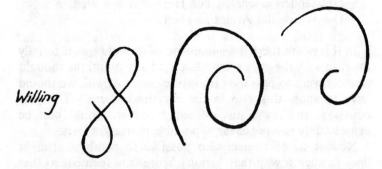

Willing

Feeling is shown by making use of some sort of combination of straight and curved lines. Here you have opportunity for a wide play of fancy.

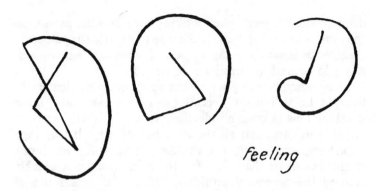

feeling

Now it will be necessary to work out eurythmy forms along these lines. All of you will be able to make such forms for yourselves, and by trying to do so you will create an inner relationship between the eurythmy and the poem. Then the question naturally arises: What is the connection between such forms as these, and those forms which have been given as standard forms, as forms which have been worked out in such a way as to bring out the special character of the poem? You will discover, however, that these guiding lines really underlie all such forms. You will invariably find this to be the case.

On the other hand, you will also find, when working out such forms, that care has been taken to show where called for, the more intimate character of a poem. What does this mean? The fact of the matter is that by far the greater number of so-called poems are in reality not poetry at all. For a true poet must be able to enter into the essential nature of language, so that what he has to say is not merely prose content more or less crudely clothed in verse, but is expressed through the way in which he handles the language itself. To express wonder in a poem by making use of some such phrase as: O how wonderful!—cannot be said to be artistic. A truly artistic sense will lead one to introduce as many *a*-sounds as possible into a poem at the moment when one most wishes to express this feeling of wonder. In the same way it would be good to make use of the *u*-sound when

107

dealing with the past, when looking back into the past. On the other hand, when there is the wish to express the gathering together of inner forces as a result of some external contact, it would be well to introduce the sound *e*.

Thus, when a true poet wishes to express the element of thought he will make special use of the *e*-sound. I am speaking now in quite an idealistic sense, for it will rarely be possible to carry out all the demands of art. If this were done very, very few poems would be written—for which one might indeed be thankful—for the poet would not quickly acquire the necessary intuition. If a poet makes use of many *e* or *i* sounds, you may be sure that he is a poet who chiefly tends to express the element of thought. He tends to the epic in poetry. Whereas you will find that a poet who is making use of the vowel sounds *a*, *o* and *u*, tends more to express feeling in his poems. A poet who makes little use of vowels and much use of consonants is one who is developing the will-side of his nature. Therefore, you must follow closely the character of the poet when building up an eurythmic form.

When, therefore, you observe that a poem arises more out of the intellect,—and this is, of course, perfectly justifiable— you will make use of straight lines in the form. When you observe that feeling is more in evidence you will combine both straight and curved lines. When, however, the element of will comes most strongly to expression in a poem, even thought coloured by feeling, then you must make use of curved lines only.

If now, bearing this in mind, you proceed to examine the various forms which have been given from time to time, you will discover, and only then can you discover, how the more intimate structure of a poem is built up and must be followed in the form.

It will perhaps be interesting to see,—paying at first no attention to its content,—what sort of result is obtained when a poem is interpreted according to the indications which have been given for *Thinking*, *Feeling* and *Willing*. One can think of poems which lend themselves to all three methods, each of which has its own particular beauty.   Let us take for example the well known poem:

Ich ging im Walde	Wandering upon a day
So für mich hin,	Through the woods alone
Um nichts zu suchen,	Following no end or purpose
Das war mein Sinn.	Letting fancy lead,—
Im Schatten sah ich	Lo, in the shade,
Ein Blümchen stehn,	I saw a little flower!
Wie Sterne leuchtend,	Shining like a star in heaven,
Wie Äuglein schön.	Lovely as a child's blue eye!

Let us in the first place interpret the poem in such a way that we bring out the *story*, that we emphasize the thought-element.   Try, therefore, to improvise a form consisting of straight lines, avoiding as far as possible all rounded movements.

Ich ging im Walde	Wandering upon a day
So für mich hin,	Through the woods alone
Um nichts zu suchen,	Following no end or purpose
Das war mein Sinn.	Letting fancy lead,—
Im Schatten sah ich	Lo, in the shade,
Ein Blümchen stehn	I saw a little flower!
Wie Sterne leuchtend,	Shining like a star in heaven
Wie Äuglein schön.	Lovely as a child's blue eye
Ich wollt' es brechen,	I made as if to pluck it
Da sagt' es fein:	But gently did it say:
Soll ich zum Welken	Shall I then be broken
Gebrochen sein?	To wither and to fade?

When the poem is expressed in this way we are left with the impression that something has been related, that we have been told something.

And now try to make a form consisting of curved lines:
Ich ging im Walde. . . .
In this case you see that the story-telling element falls completely away, and there is also nothing to represent the feeling-life.

There is, however, a strong element of feeling when, for example, the flower says: Sol ich zum Welken gebrochen sein?—or again when the poet says: Wie Sterne leuchtend, wie Äuglein schön.—Thus this poem can be expressed either according to its thinking content, its willing content, or its feeling content. Now try to make a form consisting of straight and curved lines.

Ich ging im Walde. . .

By so doing you give the impression that the poem is being inwardly experienced. Straight and curved lines together indicate that the eurythmist who is interpreting the poem continually withdraws into himself: in the case of straight lines the interpretation becomes more abstract, less apparent. And by this means the whole thing retains its inward character.

Much more is manifested outwardly when one passes over into curved lines.

Now to-day I want to speak about the significance of the colours which are to be seen on the eurythmy figures, because the study of colour in this connection will do much to deepen our whole attitude towards eurythmy.*

Here, for instance, you have in this figure an indication of the colours corresponding to the sound *a*.

Of course it is obviously impossible in our eurythmy to show the colours of all the different sounds as this has been done in the case of the eurythmy figures; for if one were to do so, one would have, for instance, when an *a* and an *o* occurred in the same line, to change, while this line was being recited, from one costume into the other. That we are not yet able to do. (We already know by experience the difficulties which arise when the costumes have to be changed between two consecutive poems. But if in the course of a poem of four verses, let us say, perhaps twenty-two or twenty-eight changes had to be effected, there would be no coping with the situation.)

* It was found that the eurythmic gestures could best be portrayed by means of figures cut out from a flat surface of wood, each one being painted with three harmonizing colours, They were carried out according to directions given by Dr. Steiner at the Goetheanum, Dornach where they may be obtained.

110

Nevertheless the colours as represented here in these figures are fundamentally true. And it is a fact that one is only able to enter right into the nature of the different sounds when one is able to experience them also as colour.

Let us consider once again the sound *a*, the sound expressing wonder, astonishment. Fundamentally speaking, colour may be said to be the external expression of our feeling-life. Our feeling-life is objectified in the outer world as colour. The reason why there is so much disagreement as to the nature of colour is that people do not observe that colour is really the external counterpart of the life of the soul.

Now to return to the feeling of amazement, of wonder. You will experience this feeling in the gesture for *a*. And you must ask yourselves: What colours are called up in me by this gesture?—Here your feelings will lead you to the colour-combination seen on this figure, blue-violet,—that is to say a combination of the so-called dark colours.

Let us, on the other hand, take *o*. The mood lying behind *o* is that of embracing something. Here you need brighter colours such as shown in the eurythmy figure for the *o*-sound.

For the reason already given it is not always possible to use these colours as they are represented here in the eurythmy figures; it will, however, be of the very greatest assistance to you if, when practising, you call up in yourselves the feeling of colour in sound, the colours for instance, of *a*, *o* or *i*, or again of *u*, which is, as we know, the expression of fear. In this way you enter by degrees into a more intimate relationship with the nature of the different movements. Thus when practising it is a good exercise to dress oneself in imagination in accordance with the colours of the eurythmy figures. This is very much to be recommended.

Picture now the colours for the sound *e*, the pale yellow combined with a certain amount of green. One feels how red and blue lose themselves in green. While with blue and violet one has the feeling of yielding oneself up, as in the case of *a* and *u*, one has, in the mood of self-assertion or of taking something into one's own being, the feeling of the lighter colours. In the *e*-sound we have the expression of being affected by something and of standing up against it. This is expressed in the green colour. Green is obtained by mixing together yellow and blue; thus by a combination of a light and a dark colour. Here we have the *e* expressed directly through the colour itself. You grow into the feeling of this gesture when you associate it with this colour.

It is quite impossible to enter into these things with the understanding; they can only be felt and experienced inwardly. For our purposes, however, we will assume that we have absorbed all this, and have come so far as to recognize that the mood of any particular sound is really represented by the corresponding eurythmy figure. Let us take the mood of the *e*-sound. One will gradually discover for oneself that whole poems are really permeated throughout with the *e*-mood. However many other vowels were to occur in such a poem, it might, nevertheless, have the *e*-mood running right through it. Take, for example, a poem, or any text which is to be expressed in eurythmy, in which, let us say, there continually occurs the feeling of being unpleasantly affected by something, but at the same time a certain resistance against what is affecting one in this way. When a poem has such a mood running through it, we shall do well to choose these colours (*e*-figure) for the dress and veil. The important thing is to learn to associate definite colours with each particular sound; then we shall gradually reach the point at which we are able to select dresses and veils suitable to a poem as a whole.

I mention all this for a very good reason, and that is to prevent the delusion arising that when a eurythmist has learned the movements for *a*, *e*, *i*, *o*, etc. there is nothing more to be done. Certainly the eurythmist may be able to *do* it all, but this by itself is no proof that he can convey it to others. You must not forget that the impression created by the eurythmic gestures is very powerful; very powerful forces are at work, although we may not be conscious of them. There is all the difference in the world between those who, in their desire to master eurythmy very rapidly,

112

would be liable to believe for instance, that the sound *i* has been made when the arm is simply held out in the right direction, and those who make the *i* in such a way that the stretched movement is clearly visible. There is a great difference whether I make the movement in this way . . . or in this way, whether I merely extend the arms or whether I bring the stretched feeling to visible expression.

In order to acquire free artistic movements while actually carrying out any gesture, it is necessary to be conscious of the feeling and mood contained in the sound in question. This, however, can only come about when one really studies the individual sounds. And an important feature of this study is the clothing of oneself in imagination in the corresponding colours. All this should be taken into account in the teaching of eurythmy, both as an art and as a means of education. Eurythmists must accustom themselves to live in the world of colour.

This experience of colour was natural to humanity in the days of the old clairvoyance, but has since been lost. It appeared again in a somewhat distorted form at the end of the Kali-Yuga in certain more or less pathological cases. And at that time one met such people who maintained that Vienna was the colour of dark lilac, Czernowitz yellow, Prague yellowish-orange. Berlin a combination of yellow and grey, Paris a shimmering of rose-colour and blue, etc., etc. At that time people were to be found who talked in this sort of fashion; and anyone possessing a feeling for such things could up to a point understand what it was that they were trying to express.

In the same way every human being has his own particular colour. This colour is of course closely connected with the astral body, which, as we know, changes with every varying emotion. Nevertheless, each individual human being may be said to possess his own fundamental colour. Thus, to the question: You were at such and such a place; what sort of people did you meet there?—one might answer: The colour of the man I saw was blue,—and another: The colour of the man I saw was red.—Such a point of view is quite justifiable.

113

It is possible to feel things in this way; for in reality it is the same impression as that which arises in the case of ordinary physical colour.

It is therefore a good exercise to call up in one's mind the connection existing between any special movement and its underlying character and colour . . . (see eurythmy figures). Here it will be of assistance to practice the sound in some such way as this. You might, for instance, take the vowel-sounds *a*, *u*, *e*, *o*, *i*, and allow the following colours to stream through the movements: blue-violet; blue-green; greenish-yellow; reddish-yellow; red-yellow-orange. You must experience the colour and make the movements simultaneously, thus working at the same time in the realm of colour and of sound. By this means the movements will become noticeably flowing and supple, and you will soon see that a certain ' style' is being developed.

This brings us to the end of to-day's lecture, and to-morrow we shall continue the study of the characteristics underlying the various aspects of the soul life.

LECTURE 7

Dornach, 2nd July 1924

The possibilities inherent in eurythmy will only be realized when the eurythmist is able to create the movements, in all their detail, out of the nature of speech itself. In eurythmy it is almost as important to have an intimate understanding of the sounds of speech as it is to have a knowledge of the actual eurythmic movements. For this reason I will show you to-day the way in which the plastic formation of speech can definitely influence eurythmy. Now the plastic, formative element is in the ordinary way not fully manifested, for it passes over into sound. It is the task of eurythmy to bring the plastic element to visible expression.

When we direct our attention to the plastic element in the sounds of speech,—and here we naturally take the consonants, for they lend themselves more particularly to plastic interpretation, imitating as they do the things and processes of the external world,—we find that the sounds divide up into four types. First we have the sounds which are quite definitely built up after the pattern of *f* or *s*; then we have the sounds of the type of *b*, *p*, *d*, or *t*. When you compare the sounds of these two groups you will find that they are completely different from one another. The *s* and *f*-sounds are formed by allowing the breath stream to be blown freely outwards. With the other sounds, *d*, *t*, *b*, *p*, the breath stream is first inwardly controlled, and it is released much more consciously; it is not blown out in this case, but thrust out. Thus we must distinguish between the ' *blowing* ' or *breath* sounds, and the ' *thrusting* ' sounds, or *sounds of force*.

The nature of these two types is therefore completely different. The breath sounds yield up, as it were, the inner

115

being of man more or less passively to the outer world. They make use of the outgoing stream of the breath in order to release the inbreathed air from the body. So that these out-breathing sounds entirely depend upon the fact that the air passes outwards.

Now this breath stream always takes to itself the form, the shape of the body. It does not, however, assert itself in the outer world, but scatters itself abroad, so that the breath sounds always have the characteristic of yielding themselves up to the world outside. It is essential to grasp the character of the breath sounds and to realize that they *yield themselves up to the outer world*. Man allows this outer world to do as it will with him; not, naturally, as regards his physical body, but as regards the form which he has transmitted to the out-going breath stream.

In the case of the consonants of force this is quite otherwise. Here we master the form given to the breath. We permeate it, as it were, with our ego; we do not permit the sound to scatter itself immediately, but compel it to retain its form for a time in the outer world. Thus in the consonants of force man appears as master in his relation to the outer world, so that here one cannot speak of a yielding oneself up to the outer world, but of an *assertion of one's own inner being*.

These two types of sound comprise the great proportion of the consonants. In reality the breath sounds express sympathy with the outer world and sounds of force sympathy with oneself. The breath sounds are free from egoism; the sounds of force are egotistical. We shall always find that when we make use of the consonants of force we do so in order to express what needs to be expressed in sharp outlines.

You know already that there is a strong plastic element in the German language. And now, bearing this in mind, let us take a word beginning with a consonant of force: Baum, *b*. You will invariably notice that a consonant of force pro-duces the effect of sharp outlines. The breath sounds, on the other hand, will never produce such outlines; they describe the reverse of everything clear-cut and definite. For instance *s* in the word: *sei* is a breath sound.

One must of course keep strictly to essentials when dealing with such matters. You will naturally be able to find any number of words which seem as though they should be expressed by means of sharp outlines, and which, nevertheless, contain breath sounds. You will, however, usually discover that there is, in such words, despite their sharp outlines, a leaning towards something indefinite, in spite of the necessity for sharp outlines which may also be present.

Now the breath sounds are: *h, ch, j, sch, s, f, w, v*. The sounds of force are: *d, t, b, p, g, k, m*, and *n*. These latter are all consonants of force, sounds which express the more egotistical attitude of soul, the assertion of one's own individual being, which one wishes to safeguard in the world outside.

Then we have a sound which lends itself particularly well to the imitation of something which is turning, which is revolving. This is the *r*-sound, which is produced by a vibration in the outgoing breath-stream. *R* is the vibrating sound.

Then we have another sound in which, when articulated rightly, the tongue must imitate a storm-tossed sea: *l*. We must make undulating movements with the tongue. *L* is the wave-sound.

When do we need these two sounds? We need them when we wish to express, not merely the merging with the outer world, nor the strengthening of the self, but something which has *movement actually inherent within it*. Movement and form are, of course, expressed both in the breath sounds and the sounds of force, but these sounds are not to the same degree an embodiment of self-contained movement as such.

When we understand the true nature of the *r*-sound, we find that it contains something which lies mid-way between the yielding up of oneself and self-assertion. The *r* expresses a certain reserve; it calls up a feeling of reserve in the spiritual and soul nature of man. For this reason we express with the *r*-sound everything which we are able to grasp and take hold of as we take hold of our own being, when forming a resolution, when making a resolve (raten).

Resolve (Rat) is a word which illustrates particularly well the special characteristic of the sound *r*. When we make a resolution we turn something over and form a judgment. This feeling of turning something over in order to make a resolution is always to be found when we enter into the nature of *r;* so that we express with words containing the sound *r* those things in the outer world which have a certain similarity to this mood of turning something over and thereby forming a judgment. Thus the *r*-sound has an egotistical quality. It does not yield up what it has created to the outer world, but retains it for itself and in itself.

And the *l* is the sound which expresses reflection, but reflection mingled with a certain yielding tendency. One would rather listen to what is said than come to a decision for oneself; one allows someone else to decide; a feeling of waiting lies in the inner experience of *l*.

Now the point is to bring the plastic nature of these sounds to actual eurythmic expression. The special characteristic of the breath sounds can best be shown in eurythmy by moving the body in such a way that the sounds are carried with it, or, in other words, by trying to follow the direction of the sounds with the body. Try, for instance, to make an *s*, moving the body in such a way that it follows in the direction of the arms as they form the sound. Make the movement for *s*, to begin with quite quietly; now make it very clearly, so that one sees that you are following the movement with the body. If the movement tends in a forwards direction, let the upper part of the body follow after it, if it tends backwards the upper part of the body must be thrown backwards also. You must have control over the whole body, and allow it to swing with the sound, to swing in the direction of the sound. Try this also with *f*, for example; let the body follow after the sound.

Now we will turn to a consonant of force. Here, too, the point is to bring the nature of the sound into the movement of the body. In this case the body must not be allowed to move, but must bring about the desired effect by means of its posture. The body must show that it intends to come to rest, to fix, as it were, the movement which is indicated by the sound. Take *b* to begin with, make it just as you like; and now stiffen yourself, stand quite still and stiffen yourself, so that one can see clearly that the sound is held. This stiffening of the body must be carried out in such a way that you actually feel it in your muscles. This inner rigidity gives to the consonants of force their special character.

It is deeply interesting to consider such things, for in the breath sounds what really comes to expression is this: I will have nothing to do with Lucifer; everything which is Luciferic must disappear.—And the consonants of force express this feeling: I will hold fast to Ahriman, for if he escapes me he will poison everything; he must be held fast. —Thus the influence of Lucifer and of Ahriman has been implanted into these sounds.

R can only be expressed fully when one tries to move the body, gently, but with a certain swing and grace, in an upward and downward direction.

In order to carry out the *l*-sound correctly there must be a free movement of the body forwards and backwards, not following the movement in this case, but showing two independent activities. When making the movement for a breath sound, the body must follow the direction of the arms; it must, as it were, accompany the movement. When making the wave-sound, the body must have an independent movement, free and rhythmic,—forwards, backwards, forwards, backwards. This rocking, which is carried out by changing the weight alternately from the heels to the toes, must be made externally visible. You will find how well you are able to do this, if you imagine that you have a rod under your feet, and see-saw, as it were, to and fro, keeping the rod— which you may picture as rolling slightly, midway between the toes and the heels. The best way to practise it is to swing so far forward that you nearly fall, only just retaining your balance,—and then to swing so far backwards that you are once more in danger of falling. If you should happen really to fall it is of no consequence; it will only serve to impress upon you the feeling of the movement.

119

If you practise the movement in this way it will gradually become habit, and you will be able to make the rocking so pronounced that you only stop at the very moment of falling. so that the onlooker would be inclined to say: How clever not to fall!—with practice such skill may be attained in the carrying out of the *l*-sound, that the onlooker is left with the impression: How clever to be able to do that without falling!

By such means you will be able really to enter into, and grasp the whole inner character of the sounds of speech.

Now we can gain a further understanding of speech and language by trying to enter into the nature of the diphthongs. The diphthongs naturally consist of a combination of two separate and essential parts. (Frl. S. . . . will you demonstrate the movement for *eu*.)*

What lies in this sound? It consists of *e* and *u*; both these sounds are contained within the *eu*, but are, as it were, left uncompleted. Try to indicate an *e* and an *u*. Stop the *e* movement just as it is being formed. What would it become if it were formed completely? We will assume for the moment that the movement has been completed. . . . But now check the movement half-way. . . . You have not yet carried it out fully, and instead of doing so must lead it over into the *u*-sound. What do we do when completely forming an *u*? The arms approach one another so closely that they actually touch. The *eu*-movement must be carried out in such a way that the arms do not merely cross one another as in the case of the *e*-sound, but lie side by side, the *definite* contact being indicated by a feeling of trying to raise the arms up towards the head. This gives you the feeling for *eu*.

Thus we begin to enter into the nature of the diphthongs. We bring together the two component parts, but in such a way that they are only suggested, not carried out completely.

This, at the same time, leads you to an understanding of a very essential characteristic of speech, of sound as such. It is in the diphthongs that you can best study the transition from

* In the German language *eu* corresponds to the English *oi* as in ' toil '.

120

one sound to the next. And at this point we must consider what kind of text is most suited to eurythmic expression. I know of an Austrian philosopher, Bartholomaus Carneri by name, who, during the last years of his life, wrote even his most difficult philosophical works in such a way that they could easily be expressed in eurythmy. This philosopher would have been driven to distraction if he had come across such a sentence as the following, for example: Lebe echte Empfindungen.—He would have thought it appalling. And why? He was simply disgusted when a word ending with a vowel was followed by another word beginning with a vowel. He asserted that such a thing should never be allowed to occur, but that wherever possible one should avoid a vowel sound at the end of one word being followed by a vowel sound at the beginning of the next. Indeed, he went so far as to write whole articles in which he endeavoured never to bring vowel-sounds into juxtaposition, but always to let the transition from one word to the next be brought about by means of the consonants.

When two vowels, or a vowel and a consonant come together, and you wish to express this in eurythmy, you will find that you have to do so by means of gentle, soft movements. On the other hand you will make the movements decided,—they will become decided by themselves,— when one word ends and the next word begins with a consonant. It is important in eurythmy really to observe what takes place when different sounds, sounds of a different character come together. This can best be studied in the diphthongs, for the diphthong is only truly brought to expression when the movement for the first sound is shown in its beginning and then led over into the latter part of the movement for the second sound.

Bearing this principle in mind, let us now form the *ei*-sound.* Let us, in the first place, make the two sounds concerned,—that is to say the *e* and *i* sounds as such. Now try not to complete the *e*-sound, but to check it as it comes into being, leading it over immediately into the final stage of

* The *ei* in the German language corresponds to the English *i* as in ' tide.'

121

the movement for *i*, In this way we have really formed the *ei*. Take as an example: ' Mein Leib ist meiner Seele Schrein.' (My body is the shrine of my soul.) Do this in such a way that you take into consideration the order of the consonants. First two sounds of force, then the ' wave ' sound, again a sound of force, then a breath sound, followed by three sounds of force, breath sound ' wave ' sound, breath sound, vibrating sound, and lastly a sound of force.

Now you must fit the *ei*-sound satisfactorily in between.

You see how these things bring movement and life into Eurythmy, but they must be really carefully studied.

Now we must try to realize the effect of the sound *ei* when it is specially strongly emphasized. (Frl. B. . . . will you show us this example): Weiden neigen weit und breit. (Willows are swaying from side to side.) You must imagine that this picture of the swaying willows has to be portrayed in paradigmatic language. (I have omitted the word ' sich '.) Thus we have *w* (English v), breath sound, then *d, n, n, g,* and again *n*, all sounds of force, again the breath sound *w*, followed by four sounds of force, *t, n, d, b*, then the vibrating sound *r* and lastly *t*, once more a sound of force.

Try now to bring all this into the sentence you are showing and those of us who are looking on must observe carefully how the characteristic *ei*-sound makes its appearance again and again. ' Weiden neigen weit und breit.'

We can take still another diphthong, the *au*.* Here again we can let the first movement merge into the second. Try to hold the movement for *a* as it first arises, thus checking it when it is about half-formed and leading it over into the *u*. Make an *a* forwards and now turn it aside before reaching the final position, finishing with the movement for *u*. When you pass over directly from the *a* to the *u*, you get the movement for *au*.

But this movement, although correct, will always lack character if we merely pass over from one sound into the other.

* The German *au* corresponds to the English *ou* as in ' ground.'

122

The effect will not be sufficiently strong. On the other hand when you carry out the movement in such a way that you begin to form the *a*-sound with one arm, at the same time bringing the other arm into contact with the body, thus forming an *u*,—when you do this, then you have a characteristic *au*. This is not the only way of making *u* (bringing the arms together), but I have also made an *u* when I simply stand up and touch the body with the left arm, bringing it slowly downwards. Try to show these words in eurythmy: Laut baut rauh.—The point here is not the sense of the words: it is simply a eurythmic exercise.

All this must of course be studied. Naturally you can make *au* in all kinds of ways; for instance, you can make it by simply bringing one arm into contact with the body (right arm in the position for *a*, left arm laid across the breast). You must try really to penetrate into the spirit of these things.

Now in order to enter further into the forms of the sounds and their connection with language, let us take the sound *ö* (as in bird). The movement is similar to the *o*, but accompanied by a spring. The *o*-movement is, as it were, torn apart. This tearing of the *o*-movement must be carried out with a certain lightness and grace,—and now add the spring. The spring must be made just as the *o*-movement is broken.

Now we will make the sound *ä*.* First make an *a* and then an *e*. Make the *a* with the legs in such a way that you step from the front backwards, at the same time making *e* with the arms. Thus you get the movement for *ä*.

There still remains the *ü*.† It is a *u*, but its special characteristic is that it is carried out with the backs of the hands laid against each other, thus indicating the *i*-sound also. You must show the *u* with the feet and at the same time you must suggest an *i* in the movement of the arms. Instead of making an *i* in this way (stretched movement), it must be shown more like this (backs of hands together, one slipping past the other). Then you have have the *ü*.

---

* This movement is made use of in English eurythmy for the sound *a* as in ' and.'
† Rudolf Steiner mentioned the word ' sweet ' as an instance in which this movement could be made use of in English eurythmy.

Take this sentence in order to see how beautiful it is when the *ü*-sounds are really brought out:

Prüfe dich, Schüler
Übe mit Mühe

(Test thyself, Pupil,
Practise with diligence.)

These words might well be taken as an eurythmist's motto:

' Prüfe dich, Schüler,
Übe mit Mühe.'

In this way we enter into the true nature of those sounds which we feel to be made up of more than one element.

What then do these diphthongs represent in language. Where do we have a diphthong, where a modified vowel? What do the diphthongs, what do the modified vowels represent in language? Wherever we have the diphthongs or modified vowels we have some such feeling as this: Now everything is becoming vague, indistinct and nebulous. This very often occurs when the singular becomes plural. For instance *one* brother (Bruder) makes a quite definite impression, but it we take the plural, that is to say, several brothers (Brüder), the feeling immediately becomes more indefinite. Thus the modified vowel represents impressions which are less sharply defined, and the same may be said with regard to the diphthongs.

If we enter into the nature of the diphthongs, we shall always find that something is present which cannot be looked upon as being entirely in the singular, but we are, as it were, given an impression of the plural, of things which are interwoven, bound together, or separated one from the other. We must always look for this in the diphthongs.

This is why in eurythmy it is so wonderful when the directly visible movements which we have for *a*, or for *i*, for example, take on in the movements for the diphthongs something of a fluidic nature, something shading off into the

124

indefinite. Eurythmy is really able to bring to expression the deepest elements of sound and language. Thus we see how the character of the individual sounds comes to visible expression in the movements of eurythmy.

Let us try the following exercise. We will ask Frau Sch. . . . and Frl. S. . . . to stand here, you (Frl. S. . . .) making the sounds *i, e, u* in succession, and you (Frau Sch. . . .) making the two remaining vowels, *a* and *o*. Now in order to show the exercise quite clearly, will you (Frl. S. . . .), make an *i*, and you (Frau Sch. . . .), follow this with an *a*, and so on, alternately, *e, o, u*. Do this in such a way that the character of the sounds is brought clearly to expression.

Let us go back to the beginning and see what it is that we are doing (Frl. S. . . . *i*, Frau Sch. . . . *a*.) The eurythmist making *i* enters right into the form of the movement, while the eurythmist making *a*, creates, as it were, the movement from outside. When Frl. S. . . . makes the *i*-sound, there is a flashing of fire, a flashing of fire outwards (this could, of course, also be done with the hand). When Frau Sch. . . . makes an *a*, she attracts to herself from without the clouds and the winds.

Frl. S. . . .
i
e
u
Frau Sch. . . .
a
o

A O apollo   IƐU Dionysos

2 4   1 3 5

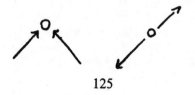

125

You see how warmth, fire lies in this sound (*i*), and how form lies in this sound (*a*). In the former you have a radiating outwards, and in the latter a plastic, form-giving element. Thus Frl. S. . . . has shown us the true Dionysos, the Dionysian vowels, and Frau Sch. . . . the true Apollo, the Apollonian vowels. This is clearly to be seen when the movements are properly carried out. So that one may say, that when a poem consists mainly of the vowels *o* and *a*, it is a plastic poem, a poem with little movement, an Apollonian poem. On the other hand, when a poem consists mainly of the vowels *i*, *u*, *e*, the fire-element is predominant; it is a Dionysian poem.

Thus you see how very much may be expressed between the lines. One has only to say to Frl. S. . . .: Make an *i* or an *e*,—and to Frau Sch. . . .: Make an *a* or an *o*,—and one has really said: You are a child of Dionysos; or: You are a child of Apollo.—In other words we may see in these vowels something of the cult of Dionysos, something of the cult of Apollo.

When one really experiences such things as these, it becomes possible, through eurythmy, to draw out in the most wonderful way the inherent characteristics of speech, and to enter into the whole being of man.

Breath Sounds: *h. sch. j. ch. s. f. v.*
   Letting oneself go with the outer world.
Sounds of Force: *d. t. b. p. g. k. m. n.*
   An assertion of one's inner being.
Vibrating Sound: *r.*
Wave Sound: *l.*

126

LECTURE 8

THE WORD AS DESCRIPTION AND THE WORD IN ITS CONTEXT

Dornach, 3rd July 1924

We must in speech eurythmy, as we have already done in tone eurythmy, differentiate between that which tends to carry the word, the tone, down into the physical world, and that which tends to raise it up into the spiritual world. We have until now paid very little attention to this difference. Yesterday, however, at the end of my lecture, I pointed out that when the vowel sound is changed into the diphthong the sense-world does not show itself in such sharply defined outlines, but appears more scattered, more diffused. And this at the same time brings us nearer to the spiritual. I pointed out that we easily see *one* brother (Bruder); when it is the case of *one*, we have a sharply defined sense-impression: whereas *several* brothers (Brüder) make a collective impression. This gathering together of individuals brings us nearer to the world of imagination, of idea, and it is this ascent into the world of idea which is expressed in the diphthong.

These diphthong sounds do indeed show themselves to be essentially of a more spiritual nature than the actual vowel-sounds of which they are composed. For just as in tone-eurythmy that which is essentially spiritual in the music does not lie in the actual tones, but between the tones, so also in speech-eurythmy, that which rays upwards to the spiritual does not lie in the sharply emphasized sound, in the sound which is uttered strongly and upon which we rest, but it lies at that point where one sound passes over into the other—thus between the sounds. For this reason the movements of eurythmy can never become really interesting as long as the eurythmist merely concentrates upon the forming of the separate sounds. But eurythmy can be made deeply interesting when one gradually learns to lead one sound over into the next. Thus we see that the truly spiritual element in eurythmic movement is brought about by the way in which one sound arises out of the other.

To this something further must be added. Fundamentally speaking every word can be looked at from two aspects. On the one hand we have the aspect of external imitation, on the other hand the placing of that which is thus expressed into the whole world order. If to-day people were more disposed to study language from a spiritual point of view, realizing the way in which each language arises from out of its own genius, great stress would be laid upon the interesting fact that, in the configuration of a word, it is not merely the individual significance of a process or thing that is described but its relationship to a collective whole. All these things must be taken into account.

Thus we must realize that, in declaiming a poem, or merely endeavouring to give a word its true proportion in a sentence, the reciter must instinctively, by means of his artistic feeling, develop this attitude towards the sounds of speech: Such or such is the relationship of a word to its whole context. I shall speak about these things in detail later. Now, however, I am trying to show how, on the one hand, words have the descriptive element, and how, on the other hand there is the possibility of going beyond the word itself and entering into the poem or sentence as a whole. We can see this best by taking definite examples. Let us first take a very characteristic type of word, the *personal pronoun*. Such words, in their very nature, place that to which they refer into some quite definite relationship, or—which is indeed much the same thing—they remove it right out of this relationship. We will take as an example the word ' ich ' (I), and ask someone to express it in eurythmy, standing still. (Frl. W. . . . will you do this?) Now, in these movements for *i* and *ch* you have expressed the word ' Ich '.

128

But to an unprejudiced observer there will be something lacking in these movements. In themselves they are quite correct, and certainly do express the word 'Ich' in visible language; and yet there is something lacking. One has the feeling that here the 'Ich' is simply represented diagrammatically; it is as if the only impression we had of a man were his portrait. Such a representation of the 'Ich' is not sufficiently living, for the spirit of man, which lies behind the manifestation of the 'Ich', is not fully expressed. What then is the spiritual essence of the word 'Ich'? In this word there lies the pointing back to oneself, the concept of the self, but the concept of the self turned inwards towards the self. And if one wishes to express this backward turning into the self, it can be done excellently, not by standing still, but by moving. Let us suppose, therefore, that you take two steps forwards and then two steps backwards, forwards, backwards, forwards, backwards.

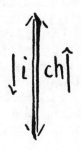

Thus you will retrace your steps, going back over the same line and returning to your starting point. With the two forward steps do the *i*-sound, and with the two backward steps the *ch*. In this way movement enters into the expression of the word 'Ich', movement, which finds its way back again into itself just as the 'Ich' conception contains the feeling of turning back into the self.

If you carry out the movements in this way, taking two steps forwards with the *i*, and two steps backwards with the

129

ch, you will enter right into the form (see diagram), and this form is of such a nature that it grows directly out of the meaning inherent in this combination of sounds.

Let us pass over from the 'Ich' (I) to the 'Du' (Thou). Here we have quite another feeling. The whole relationship is different, indicating a connection with some other being. (Frl. S. . . . will you make the movements for 'Du', standing still as before: *d-u*?) But in this simple expression of the 'Du' there is again a certain feeling of dissatisfaction, for here again we only have the picture of the 'Du', not ,the actual 'Du' itself. The movement is not living. The real spirit of the word is lacking. We must seek some means which will help us to find our way to this spirit.

In the case of the word 'Ich' it is quite clear that one turns back into oneself. With the word 'Du'—when one really enters into the nature of the 'Du', thus coming into contact with somebody not oneself, *the other*,—then one goes out of oneself. Here one cannot go back on the same line and touch the starting point again, for this would lead one back into oneself. That is obviously impossible. On the other hand, one cannot go altogether out of oneself, for then one would not be expressing the word 'Du', but the word 'Er' or 'Sie' (He or She). You will easily feel this. Thus with 'Du' it is necessary to give some slight indication of one's own being also. This can only be done when the line of the form turns back, touching itself at some definite point.

This diagram shows the point at which you cross your previous line. When, therefore, instead of simply going forwards and backwards, you only touch the line of the form once on your way back, you have the complete movement for 'Du'. The *d* should be made during the first part of the form, and the *u* on the way back; but the line must only cross itself at the one point. Now you have really brought the 'Du' into movement, and have done so in such a way that it has not become an 'Er' or a 'Sie'. You have retained a certain contact with yourself, even if this contact is but slight. It is, however, possible to strengthen the feeling of oneself. If we wish to do this, if we wish the going out from ourselves to become weaker and weaker, then, while making the *u*, the form can be carried out in this way:

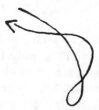

This 'Du' would, however, in no way express a loving feeling. If you try the form for yourself you will notice that the effect is somewhat pinched, much less out-going in character. Such things as these can, of course, only be realized through the feelings; they are, however, not difficult to feel.

I have already indicated the way in which the 'Er' can be shown. The impression of 'Er' is given by never allowing the second part of the form to touch the line taken by the first part of the form. Thus we find that the 'Er' form is the circle, where we have a line which is never touched again until the starting point is reached. The 'Er' must be expressed by a circular form, by a line which never turns back on to itself.

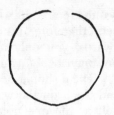

Here we have another possibility.

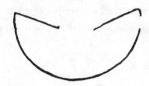

You do not come back to your starting point, and, were you to do so, the form would already be completed. Thus we have a line which never crosses itself at any point, and which expresses for us the word ' Er '. (Frl. S. . . . will you come and make the movements for ' Er ' standing still?) It is impossible to give the real feeling for ' Er ' while standing still; one cannot even produce a pictorial impression. All that we have is the egotistical contemplation of the other person or thing. There is no going out of oneself. Now add this form to the movements; simply make a circle, so that you come back to the point from which you started. Accompany one side of the form with the *e* and the other side with the *r*, and you will see how well the feeling of the ' Er ' is expressed.

Some time ago I gave an exercise built up upon a special combination of sounds. It began with the word ' Der ' (The), which is indeed similar in character to ' Er '; and it was built up on the ' Er ' feeling and carried out in such a way that the form never at any point came back and touched the previous line. (Frau Sch. . . . will you show us

this exercise, ' Der Wolkendurchleuchter '; try and do it
in such a way that you bring into it all that I have said.)

> Der Wolkendurchleuchter,
> Er durchleuchte,
> Er durchsonne,
> Er durchglühe,
> Er durchwärme
> Auch mich.

> (He who illuminates the clouds,
> May he illuminate,
> May he irradiate,
> May he inspire
> And fill with warmth and light,
> Even me.)

She has now done this in such a way that the character of
' Er ', (He) upon which the entire poem is built, was
shown in the exercise as a whole. She has done it in such a
way that the ' Er ' was carried in movement through the
whole poem. There is, however, another way of doing
the exercise. Every time the word ' Er ', (He) occurs,
make a circle; but also carry out the form of a circle in the
course of the whole poem. Thus, whenever the word
' Er ' appears make a circle, go a little further, make another
circle, and so on. By this means the whole thing takes on
a quite different character, quite another type of movement.

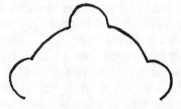

In the old way of doing this exercise we felt that we must
devote ourselves more to the *mood of the poem as a whole.*

In the new way we give ourselves up to the changing moods, to the illuminating, the irradiating, the inspiring with warmth and light.

Passing over from the 'Ich' (I) to the 'Wir' (We), that is to say from the singular to the plural,—for 'We' implies at least two people,—we are no longer dealing with a solo-dance, but have come into the realm of the round dance. If there are two people taking part in the form, it can be done in the following way (see diagram). The working together, the losing of the self, is expressed by means of the circle. The 'Ich' is expressed by each individual taking a number of steps forward and at the same time saying aloud the word 'Wir' or 'We', and then going back over the same line,—forwards, backwards, forwards, backwards. In this way the two aspects of the word are shown quite clearly. Thus, if only two people are taking part, they stand opposite to one another, approach each other, draw back again, approach each other, draw back again, and in so doing express the inner feeling of the word 'Wir'.

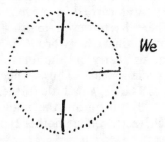

We

If four people take part the circle becomes more complete, and by moving forwards and backwards over the same line the 'Wir' is very well expressed. The feeling of belonging together can be strengthened by taking hands, but this will hardly be possible with two people only. Here we have a very beautiful expression of 'Wir'. Let four eurythmists stand in a circle, saying the word 'Wir' or 'We' aloud, in the way I have already explained. Begin by joining hands; now take two steps forwards with the *w*, passing over into the *i* when you have reached the centre; complete the backward journey with *r*, and again join hands. Care must be taken not to make the *i* too soon. In this way we really express the word ' Wir '. Quite beautiful shades of feeling can be brought into such an exercise. One must, however, always experience the difference between ' Ich ', ' Wir ', and so on.

There is still another exercise which can be very beautiful. If four eurythmists stand as indicated in the diagram, not taking hands this time, but making the movements backwards, what will this express?—' Ihr ' (You). We have ' Du ' (Thou) carried over into the plural. There can be no doubt about it; it is quite apparent. In this exercise we show the turning away from ourselves, the feeling of ' Ihr '.

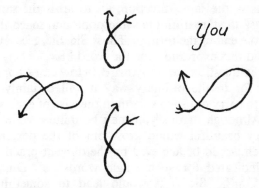

The word ' Ihr ' must also be spoken aloud. And from the very beginning the arms must tend in a backward direction. In this way much that is of significance can be brought into the exercise. These things should also be taken into account when studying the structure of a poem, for they are exceedingly characteristic. All that can be felt and experienced in the single words, particularly in such characteristic words as the personal pronouns, must be sought for and experienced in the structure of language as a whole. Very much more could be said on this subject, but for the moment we will pass on to another exercise.

Let us ask three eurythmists to place themselves in a triangle, and then carry out this form:

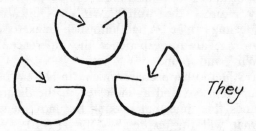

Here you have ' Sie ' (They), the plural of ' Er '.

If you wish to give characteristic expression to the word ' Sie ', you will do so most easily when you all three move the forms in the same direction, all towards the same side. (You must all start from the same point and reach the same point at the end of the form.) Thus: Sie, Sie, Sie. Here we have the direct expression for the word ' Sie,'.

Now the question naturally arises: How can I apply these things?—for in the ordinary way it will certainly not be possible to carry out such a form in the case of each separate word. Although of this you may be quite certain—something very beautiful would grow out of the dexterity and skill which would be achieved by the diligent practice of all I have indicated for such single words as ' Du ', ' Er ', ' Wir ', ' Ihr ', ' Sie '. It would lead to something very beautiful.

In the case of certain poems we have quite definitely the ' Ich ' or ' I ' character. In other poems, especially in love poems, we have the ' Du ' or ' Thou ' character. And in the case of quite a number of poems,—here I am reminded particularly of nearly all the poems of Martin Greif,—we have a most pronounced ' Er ' or ' He ' character. One can enter right into the whole mood of a poem when one is able to perceive in a poem itself the ' I ', ' Thou ' or ' He ' character, and then express the poem by means of a form which has been drawn from out of the

136

very nature of the 'I', 'Thou', 'He', 'We', 'You', or 'They'. A specially beautiful effect may be attained, when the objective mood, the mood of 'He', the mood of going out of oneself, is carried over into what is more subjective in its feeling. Let us take as an example that poem from which we have learned so much already, for from whichever point of view we look at it, it seems as if specially written for the study of eurythmy. I refer to Goethe's famous poem so well known to us all:

> Über allen Gipfeln
> Ist Ruh;
> In allen Wipfeln
> Spürest du
> Kaum einen Hauch;
> Die Vögelein schweigen im Walde.
> Warte nur, balde
> Ruhest du auch.

> (O'er all the hill tops
> Is quiet now;
> In all the tree tops
> Hearest thou
> Hardly a breath;
> The birds are asleep in the trees
> Wait, soon like these
> Thou too shalt rest.)

Let us analyse this poem quite objectively:

> Über allen Gipfeln
> Ist Ruh.

We will give this the 'He' character.

> In allen Wipfeln
> Spürest du
> Kaum einen Hauch;

137

Here we pass on to the 'Thou'.

> Die Vögelein schweigen im Walde.   Er. (He)
> Warte nur, balde
> Ruhest du auch.

Now we must ask: Should this be in the 'I' or the 'Thou' character? For Goethe is here speaking to himself. You could try it both ways. Let us first try it in this way:

> Über allen Gipfeln
> Ist Ruh;   Er. (He)
> In allen Wipfeln
> Spürest du
> Kaum einen Hauch;   Du. (Thou)
> Die Vögelein schweigen im Walde Er. (He)
> Warte nur, balde
> Ruhest du auch.   Du. (Thou)

If we do so we shall see how the form arises out of the whole mood of the poem. Personal pronouns, such as 'Ich', 'Du' and so on, are, when uttered, in reality nothing else than a crystallization, a condensation of a mood or feeling otherwise spread over a whole passage. In this particular poem the first lines are permeated by the 'He' mood, the next lines by the 'Thou', then comes the 'He' once more, then again the 'Thou', or, as we shall presently see, the 'I', which is the mood of the last lines.

> Warte nur, balde
> Ruhest du auch.

Now let us do the whole poem in this second way: He, Thou, He, I:

> Über allen Gipfeln
> Ist Ruh;   Er. (He)
> In allen Wipfeln

138

Spürest du
Kaum einen Hauch;   Du. (Thou)
Die Vögelein schweigen im Walde. Er. (He)
Warte nur, balde
Ruhest du auch.   Ich.(I).

Now, by giving the form the ' I ' character, you have
seen how entirely different it becomes. If we try both
forms one after the other, we shall certainly decide that the
second is the better. This will undoubtedly prove to be the
right way. From such a poem you can gain the most
wonderful perception of how the form develops right out
of the poem itself. You must learn to feel the relationship
existing between a certain combination of sounds and the
meaning of the word thus formed—a personal pronoun, for
example.

Consider for a moment how beautifully some such short
poem as the following can be worked out, if we study its
meaning and make use of all that we now know:

Schlummer und Schlaf, zwei Brüder, zum Dienste der
    Götter berufen,
Bat sich Prometheus herab, seinem Geschlechte zum Trost.
Aber den Göttern so leicht, doch schwer zu ertragen den
    Menschen,
Ward nun ihr Schlummer uns Schlaf, ward nun ihr Schlaf
    uns zum Tod.

Here the word ' Uns ' (Us) occurs twice; we will, of
course, treat it in the same way as ' Wir—' (We), and make
use of the ' Wir ' form. If we now look more closely into
the poem, we shall be able to analyse it as follows:

Schlummer und Schlaf, zwei Brüder, zum Dienste der Götter
    berufen.

Obviously an ' Er ' form.

Bat sich Prometheus herab, seinem Geschlechte zum Trost.

Now in the word 'Bitten' (to ask) there is necessarily a turning towards some other person, there is an indication of the 'Du'; we feel the underlying character of 'Du'.

Aber den Göttern so leicht, doch schwer zu ertragen den
     Menschen.

With these words we pass over to something which leads us into the depths of our own being. Such knowledge can only be attained by entering into the very nature of the thing in question. Here, therefore, an opportunity presents itself of making use of the position I have already shown you, the position for *Knowledge*.

Ward nun ihr Schlummer uns Schlaf.

The light sleep of the Gods becomes deep sleep for man, and the deep sleep of the Gods becomes death for man.

Ward nun ihr Schlaf uns zum Tod.

Here we come into the region of destiny, common to all men by reason of their humanity; we have the 'Wir'. We shall be able to make a form which really brings life into the poem if we make use, in the first place, of those forms which we have gained from a study of the personal pronouns, and, in the second place,—where the whole thing is brought into the realm of the spiritual,—of the movement, the position for *Knowledge*. We shall get good results if we regard these forms as really fundamental forms, and make use of them quite freely, but with due regard to the sense and correctness of the way in which they are applied.

Frl. S. . . . will you do the first line to an 'Er' form, fitting in the whole line to the one form. With the second line make a 'Du' form. With the third, or rather in the pause between the second and third lines, and again at the end of the third line, take up the position for *Knowledge*, finally using the ' Wir ' form for the last line. You will, however, not be able to make the ' Wir ' form alone; two other eurythmists must, therefore, make their appearance on the stage, one coming from the left wing, the other from the right. By this means the last line will be coloured with the feeling of ' Wir ', of 'We '. This example shows you how such forms may be worked out. They are developed from out of the poems themselves.

From all that has been said, and from these simple examples, I hope you are beginning to understand the spirit in which the study of eurythmy has to be undertaken. With eurythmy one has really to *study* the poem; it is not enough merely to learn the sounds, but one must enter right into its whole content, into all the nuances of feeling and fine shades of mood contained within it. And no one should attempt to express a poem in eurythmy, who has not first put to himself the question: What is the fundamental character of this poem?—upon what artistic foundation is it based?

Let us take another example from Goethe:

Seid, o Geister des Hains, o seid, ihr Nymphen des Flusses,
     Eurer Entfernten gedenk, euer Nahen zur Lust!
Weihend feierten sie im stillen die ländlichen Feste;
     Wir, dem gebahnten Pfad folgend, beschleichen das
          Glück.
Amor wohne mit uns; es macht der himmlische Knabe
     Gegenwärtige lieb und die Entfernten euch nah.

Now as a preliminary study we must begin carefully to examine the poem. These things, which I am necessarily treating in a somewhat sketchy way at the moment, must be gone into thoroughly and in detail when one is working out a poem with a view to doing it in eurythmy.

So we have:

Seid, o Geister des Hains, o seid, ihr Nymphen des Flusses.

141

What is this but the ' Du ' mood, a form of address. If you are working out the poem with several eurythmists, as we mean to do now, you will, of course, begin with the ' Ihr ' form.

Eurer Entfernten gedenk, euern Nahen zur Lust!
Once more ' Ihr '.
Weihend feierten sie im stillen die ländlichen Feste; ' Sie '.
Wir, dem gebahnten Pfad folgend, beschleichen das
    Glück.   ' Wir '.
Amor wohne mit uns, es macht der himmlische Knabe.
    ' Er '.
Gegenwärtige lieb und die Entfernten euch nah.   ' Ihr'.

In the second line we repeat the ' Ihr ' form, in order to express ' Euch ' (your). The example consists of six lines.

I will now ask three eurythmists to group themselves together and express the whole poem in the way I have indicated. Before beginning you must be quite clear about what it is you have to do. You must make the form according to the rules given. In this case, therefore, ' Ihr ', ' Ihr ', ' Sie ', ' Wir ', ' Er ', ' Ihr ',—each form to spread out over a whole line.

There are, of course, other ways of doing it. Two of the eurythmists can remain standing, and the third do the ' Er' form alone; then we should have:

Amor wohne mit uns; es macht der himmlische Knabe—

done as a solo line, after which all three would join together in the ' Ihr ' form.

Gegenwärtige lieb und die Enfernten euch nah.

In this way we learn to realize the possibility of studying a poem by means of the eurythmic forms.

LECTURE 9

Dornach, 4th July 1924

To-day we will consider certain things bound up with the plastic element of speech, with a method of speaking which gradually leads over into the realm of art. When doing eurythmy,—it is well to be clear on this point,—we can either do the movements standing still or accompanied by walking. We have already seen the significance of eurythmic walking.

Walking is, fundamentally speaking, the expression of an impulse of will. When studying eurythmy it is essential to understand the inner nature of all that is bound up with speech, and, consequently, with visible speech also. When taking a step we can clearly differentiate three separate phases: 1. The lifting of the foot. 2. The carrying of the foot. 3. The placing of the foot. We must be conscious that in these three phases a whole event can come to expression. First we have the raising of the foot. Then the foot remains for a moment in the air, it is carried; thus the second phase is the carrying of the foot. And finally, in the third phase, the foot is placed on the ground.

Naturally, when walking in ordinary life, it is not necessary to bother about these details. In eurythmy, however, everything must become conscious.

Thus we have:

1. The Lifting of the Foot.
2. The Carrying of the Foot.
3. The Placing of the Foot.

It is clear that much variety can be introduced by means of the different ways in which these three phases of walking are carried out.

If, in the first place, we take the lifting of the foot, we see that this clearly indicates the will-impulse inherent in the action of walking: thus with the lifting of the foot we have to do with an impulse of will. When, on the other hand, we direct our attention to the carrying of the foot, we have to do with the thought element which lies behind every will activity.

In the first place, then, we have to do with the will-impulse as such. Secondly, with the carrying of the foot, we have to do with the thought which comes to expression in this will-impulse. And in the placing of the foot the act of will is completed; here we have the deed.

1. The Lifting: Impulse of Will
2. The Carrying: Thought
3. The Placing: Deed

Now much variety can be brought into walking by making the middle phase of longer or shorter duration, also by actually making the step itself longer or shorter. Thus, the laying stress upon the middle phase of the step mainly serves the purpose of emphasizing and bringing to expression the thought which lies behind the impulse of will; it gives form to this thought.

On the other hand, by the way in which the foot is placed upon the ground, you can always show whether you think the will-impulse has achieved its goal, or whether it has faltered in its purpose. If you put your foot down uncertainly, as though walking on thin ice, your step will express uncertainty of purpose. If you put your foot down firmly, with the assurance that the ground will not give way under your feet, you will show that your goal is sure and certain.

Here, too, when working out a poem, you must analyse carefully and ask yourself whether the one mood or the other predominates. Of course such things as these only become really clear when they are practically applied. Now, however, we will pass on to other aspects of walking. And this brings us into the domain of *rhythmic walking*, into that poetic element which must enter into eurythmy, into the movements and forms of eurythmy.

It is indeed above all things important to realize consciously that, either through special emphasis, or through the longer and shorter syllables, rhythm must be brought into speech. And this rhythm must also make its appearance when expressing a poem in eurythmy. For it would have been impossible to call this art of movement of which we are now speaking 'Eurythmy', if we had not taken into account the element of rhythm.

This leads us over to a fact which must be considered if we are really to enter into the nature of speech eurythmy,— a fact that is deeply impressed into all that is connected with the more artistic aspect of speech. We have, within our modern civilization, two types of language,—prose and poetry. The further we go back in human evolution, the more we find that poetical language is really the only language, and that the human being when speaking has the longing to bring into his speech the element of poetry, the artistic element. Speech may really be said to lie midway between thinking and feeling. Thinking lies on the one side, feeling on the other. As human beings we have the inward experience of both thought and feeling. And when we express ourselves outwardly, when we try to bring something to external expression in speech, we really place speech midway between the two elements of thought and feeling.

Thought

Speech

Feeling

In the earlier periods of evolution man had an inner life of feeling somewhat different from ours to-day. The man of earlier times always had the longing, when feeling something deeply, when experiencing feeling in his soul, also to experience words rising up within him,—words which were not so clear cut and definite as our words are to-day, but which were, nevertheless, of the nature of articulated tones. He was able, as it were, inwardly to hear that which he experienced as feeling.

145

The thinking of primitive man was also different from our thinking to-day; he really thought in words. These words, however, in which he *thought* were more definite than those in which he *felt*. Thus words resounded within him. His was not such an abstract thinking as ours to-day; and words also resounded within him when he experienced feeling. That absolutely inward feeling which we possess and which has no need of words was not present in his soul. Now when we consider how closely the primitive life of the soul was bound up with word-configuration, with tone-configuration, we shall realize that an inner recitation,—if I may so describe it,—lay, in those early times, behind the thinking and feeling of man, a recitation based upon the combined development of speech, thinking and feeling. And this inner recitation differentiated itself, becoming on the one side speech which retained its artistic element, and on the other side music, that which is purely musical, the wordless sounding of tones which depends for its effect upon pitch, and so on. I dealt with this latter aspect in the course of lectures on tone-eurythmy.*

But yet another differentiation took place,—the development of pure thought. And to-day I shall speak of the essential difference between these two types of language, between poetic language which must be given artistic shape and form, and prose language, which depends entirely upon the intellectual content, and where there is no longer any necessity to give artistic form to the language as such.

During the course of the last few centuries, as materialistic thought developed—(for the abstract thought of materialism is closely bound up with the prose element)—the true feeling for the artistic shaping and forming of language was lost. And to-day we find any number of people having absolutely no feeling for the *artistic, plastic* element of language. They only regard language as a medium for the expression of thought, and are quite indifferent to the quality of the language through which this thought is expressed.

I should not enter into all these things so fully if they were

---

* Eurythmie als sichbarer Gesang.

not of the deepest significance for the understanding of eurythmy. For, in speaking about eurythmy, and taking the sounds as our starting point, we must enter at once into the realm of art. We must bring the *inner soul-nature* of the sounds to outward expression; we must, as it were, go back to a time in which man felt in the word itself all that he experienced in his soul as sound, to a time in which there really was a true language of sound. To-day there is no longer a *true language of sound*. We have instead an *intellectualistic* language which only serves to express concepts and thoughts. And this is the reason why to-day in recitation and declamation people no longer perceive the artistic, plastic element in language, the musical element, the form-giving element, but make the mistake of looking only for the meaning, of emphasizing the meaning, which is, of course, also present in prose.

It is essential for every eurythmist to gain a true perception of the difference between poetic or artistic language and the language of prose. For the mere understanding, it is, of course, a matter of no importance as to whether the wording of an idea is beautiful or ugly, as to whether or no words create a noble impression. But for an artistic forming and shaping of speech it is just these shades of feeling and character which are so important. And this is why we must strive to gain an understanding of the *artistic, plastic formation of language*.

The first step towards this understanding is the development of an inner feeling for the Iambic and Trochaic rhythms. For the moment we will not bother as to whether we will express the Iambic measure by a strongly emphasized beat preceded by one less strongly emphasized, or whether we will show it by a long beat preceded by a short beat. I shall speak of these details—which really belong more to the essential difference between recitation and declamation—in a later lecture. We must feel to begin with the real significance of starting with an unemphasized syllable and following this by an emphasized syllable, and the way in which such a rhythm carries us forwards.

147

'Auf Bergen flammen Feuer.'

Here we have an unemphasized syllable followed by an emphasized syllable. This is repeated three times, the fourth time being incomplete. We pass over from the quieter to that which has more movement, from the weaker to the stronger. This brings into walking a special characteristic, the characteristic of going towards something, the wish to reach something. And when we step to this rhythm we feel immediately that we enter into the inner element of the *will*. The Iambic element brings into speech the character of will.

Let us now take the opposite. Here the emphasized syllable occurs first, followed by the unemphasized syllable.

' Trag mir Wasser herab.'

This is just the reverse of the previous example. We begin with the strong, important beat, and pass over to the weaker, less accented beat. If you move in such a rhythm and enter into its feeling, you will at once perceive that here one takes one's start from something quite definite. And this feeling of something quite definite can only be present when you have a clear concept, a clear-cut *thought*. In this case you do not strive towards something, but you express in the rhythm your definite thoughts. Thus with the Trochaic rhythm we have to do with thinking. This thinking naturally manifests itself in action, but thought is really the dominant factor.

Will, striving, predominates in the Iambic measure; thought, the realization of thought in the Trochaic measure. You must not, of course, carry these indications to extremes. You might, for instance, picture this energetic Iambic rhythm as being expressed by a rapid progress downhill, and connect this progress with an activity of will. On the other hand you will be more inclined to connect the Trochaic rhythm with ' seeing ' or perception. As I said, you must not carry such things to extremes, but if you really enter into the nature of the different rhythms, you will find what I have said to be correct.

Now the point is to bring the Iambic and Trochaic rhythms into walking. This has, of course, already been practised. (Frl. S. . . . will you first show us the Iambic rhythm.)

And now, in order to illustrate the contrast, will you step to ' Trag mir Wasser herab ', strongly emphasizing the first beat. We must remember that with the unaccented beat we simply step, whereas with the accented beat the placing of the foot on the ground must be strongly marked. How must the foot be placed on the ground? The toes must touch the ground first, the other part of the foot following. It is quite time for eurythmists to be able to do this really as it should be done. The normal walking must be carried out in such a way that *the toes touch the ground first* the rest of the foot following after. Eurythmists must not simply trip along on their toes, but really place the whole foot on the ground.

Here are two examples.

U   —   U   —   U   —   U

Auf Bergen flammen Feuer.

—   U   —   U   —   U

Trag mir Wasser herab.

I can easily show you, by taking a more complicated rhythm, that these things really are of importance. Instead of expressing the yearning, the will, the desire in such a way that we show that we are sure of instantly achieving our object, we can prolong the feeling of desire by having two short beats, followed by a long beat. In this way we get the Anapestic rhythm:

UU   —   UU   —   UU   —

Now anyone who walks to a poem in Anapestic rhythm, and compares this with the experience of Iambic walking will notice a tremendous difference between the two. Let us take the following as an example of the Anapest:

149

Von mir bist du zum Menschen gebildet.

U U — U U — U U — U

Here there is the feeling of reaching the accented syllable with more difficulty.   This feeling of difficulty brings a more intimate character into language.   And this intimacy of character brings with it a more spiritual element.   Thus we may say that the Anapest rhythm introduces into language a certain inwardness of feeling, a certain spirituality.

(Frl. S. . . . will you show us the Anapest rhythm:)

Von mir bist du zum Menschen gebildet.

This is a perfectly clear Anapest.

Now in eurythmy the point is not so much that one hears the rhythm, but that one should be able to *see* it; for eurythmy is *visible speech*.   And for this it is necessary to accustom oneself clearly to show the emphasis on the strong beat, then the unaccented beat will take care of itself.   And it may be said that one only enters into the sphere of eurythmy when these rhythms are accompanied by an upward and downward movement of the body.

When we make the opposite rhythm, the Trochaic, a little more complicated, we get the Dactyl: long, short, short, long, short, short.   Let us take the following as an example:

Sing mir, unsterbliche Seele, der sündigen Menschen Erlösung

—   U U — U U — U U — U U —   U U — U

Try now to walk in the Dactyl rhythm and you will find that this has more the feeling of a statement, an assertion. If, however, you wish to show the true character of the Dactyl, you must not allow the body to have a forward tendency.   In this rhythm the body should remain somewhat behind.

In the rhythms we have the *time-element;* the time-element is in this way brought to eurythmic expression.   And the possibilities of eurythmy are so great just because the eurythmist is able to make simultaneous use of both *time*, and *space*.   It is possible,—to some extent even with one

150

eurythmist, but with a group much more so,—to bring into eurythmy all manner of variations of forms by means of symmetry, by the grouping of the people in some special form and by the symmetrical movement of the arms and legs. The solo eurythmist also can create forms in space, but the effect of group forms is much more powerful. The possibilities of group forms are infinitely greater.

By means of such forms, by means of this working in space, one is able to enter into the poetic element of speech even more easily, more unhampered, than is possible in recitation and declamation. Truly, recitation and declamation must also work towards the inner artistic element inherent in speech, but here the difficulties are greater than in the case of eurythmy.

The essential thing about prose language is that it enables one clearly to understand and grasp what one wishes to express by means of a word or sentence. At least one must believe one has grasped it. In prose language we have become so extreme in our desire for clarity that we make use of the so-called definition. There is really something appalling about definitions, for they make people believe that they have clearly expressed some idea, whereas, in reality, the description is merely pedantic. If people are themselves not clear about the meaning of a word, definitions will be of no help to them. In any case a comprehensive definition, even of a relatively simple thing, would necessarily lead one into endless complication; otherwise the results would be similar to the story that I have so often repeated, in which somebody described the human being as a two-legged creature without feathers. On the following day this person was confronted with a goose and told that, according to his definition, the goose was a human being, for it had two legs and no feathers—(you see, it was a plucked goose!). Now a human being is not *always* a goose, so here the definition did not meet the case.

When using prose language, one should at least attempt to express one's ideas directly, in clear outline. This way of speaking cannot—and need not—be retained in the artistic

151

formation of language . An artistic treatment of language demands imagination and fantasy; and here one should strive to use one's gift of fantasy, to give rein to one's imagination. This, however, can only be attained when one does not rest content with crude description, but when one develops an attitude of mind which allows imagination and fantasy to give form and life to whatever may be in question. If anyone were to say, for instance: ' Here is a water lily,' he would be speaking prose. But if he were to say: ' O flowering swan! ' this would be pictorial, poetical. One can quite well picture a water lily, with its white bloom rising out of the water, as a flowering swan.

The picture can also be reversed—and here I will quote from Geibel. The lines in which he describes the swan as a floating water lily are perhaps the most beautiful he has written:

> O Wasserrose, du blühender Schwan,
> O Schwan, du schwimmende Rose. ... .
> (O water lily, thou flowering swan,
> O swan, thou floating lily. . . .)

Even this can hardly be said to be an adequate picture, but at any rate it brings us much nearer to the truth.

Now how does this picture of the ' flowering swan ' arise? —The expression ' flowering swan ' is only an image; it is not in accordance with reality. A picture must have this quality; it must make us feel that it goes beyond reality and give us an impression which transcends its own imagery. The fact that a swan is not a blossom makes the expression ' flowering swan ' into a picture. It is when we feel that there is something suggestive about the picture that we are brought closer to the true nature of that which is being described.

The inner plastic element of language depends upon this possibility of imagery. And you, my dear friends, will be able to discover this pictorial element when you realize that a sound is, in itself, always a picture. A sound is no less a picture of what it describes than this expression of the

' flowering swan ' is a picture of the water lily. For the connection between the sound and what it represents does not rest on an abstraction but on life itself.

Thus it may be said that the use of language is based upon the fact that every sound is a picture, an image of what it wishes to describe. If then, we accustom ourselves to see pictures in sounds we shall learn by degrees to have a feeling for the use of these pictures,—we shall learn to know that poetic language, artistic, plastic language, must be pictorial in character.

Now, when I say: ' O flowering swan ', when meaning a water lily, and: ' O floating flower ', when meaning a swan, these two conceptions have really only one characteristic in common,—their dazzling whiteness. Their other qualities are different.

It is not difficult to form such pictures as these. They generally go by the name of metaphor. A metaphor is, in reality, a picture which makes use of some common characteristic or characteristics in order to experience what two things to be portrayed have in common. In such a case one portrays one thing by describing it as something else which is not the thing to which one is really referring, but has certain characteristics in common with it. Metaphor arises in this way.

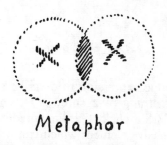

Metaphor

I am purposely not giving the usual definition of the metaphor, for this definition has nothing artistic about it. My description is not based upon logic, but I have tried to build it up from what is really essential.

153

Let us go a little further. It is possible, by making use of a word which represents something less comprehensive to express something really wider in its meaning. For instance, one can *mean* ' beasts of prey ', but if one wishes to be more pictorial, instead of actually using this expression, one might equally well say: ' the lions '. When, in using the word ' lion ', one really intends to convey the meaning of ' beasts of prey ', language becomes pictorial. We must be clear that in such a case the lesser is used to describe the greater. We wish to give the impression of what is more comprehensive, but in order to do so we use a word which expresses something more limited. This pictorial means of expression is very general. It is called the Synecdoche. In the Synecdoche we have a picture in which one makes use of the lesser to express the greater.

The reverse is also possible; it is possible to make use of the greater to express the lesser. A particularly strong impression is created by this means. For instance we have

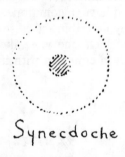

Synecdoche

Byron's picturesque expression to describe the attitude of a lady who is something of a shrew. He says: ' She looks curtain-lectures ' (Sie blickt Gardinenpredigten). Here you have a comprehensive element which can otherwise only be verbally indicated by such expressions as ' curtain-lectures ' and so on, applied to the narrower sphere of the lady's look. It is a wonderfully effective figure of speech, when the facial expression of the worst kind of Xanthippe is characterized by applying to her look the entire series of curtain-lectures with

154

all the abuse and scolding and outcry they involve. In this case the more comprehensive is used for the more limited.

We must find a means of expressing these things in eurythmy. First let us try in the simplest way. Wherever a metaphor occurs it may be shown by taking a step sideways, —either towards the right or towards the left. Wherever you have to do with anything in the nature of a metaphor you may introduce this sideways movement into the form.

If you wish to express the Synecdoche in a case where the greater is used to express the lesser, you must go backwards; if, on the other hand, you use the lesser to express the greater you must go forwards. This lies in the form. Therefore you will always express: ' She looks curtain-lectures ' by moving in a backward direction; you will, however, move forwards when, meaning ' beasts of prey ', you simply use the word ' lion '. If therefore in eurythmy you move backwards in space you immediately give the impression of reaching towards something more comprehensive, whereas moving forwards signifies entering into something less comprehensive.

In order to illustrate this, try to express by means of the direction in which you move, the following sentence:

' I strive towards the heavenly powers '

(moving backwards)

And now I shall immediately take another example, so that you may see the difference between the two:

' I shut myself within my little room '

(moving forwards)

You must express these examples simply by means of the direction in which you move. With the first, which indicates a striving towards the greater, you must go backwards. With the second: ' I shut myself within my little room ' you must go forwards. In this way we have the possibility of expressing, by means of a forwards and backwards movement, all the inner shades of feeling contained in these things.

What I have here indicated is of the utmost importance for stage art in general. For only by understanding the meaning of this walking in a forwards, backwards or sideways direction, does one learn to move on the stage in the right way. Without such understanding one might quite well try to express something of the nature of a prayer by means of a forwards-moving line, which would be utterly out of place, for in the case of a prayer or a petition the backwards-moving one at once gives the right feeling. When expressing the wish to teach something, thus entering into the realm of thought, one will not go backwards, but forwards in the form.

In the case of a conversation, the movement is neither backwards nor forwards, but sideways; for conversation is really of the nature of metaphor.

To-day I have indicated several things which, as they are further developed, will serve to make speech eurythmy more complete and worthy of being called an art in the true sense.

LECTURE 10

Dornach, 7th July 1924

Up to this point we have, at least to some extent, derived the eurythmic gestures from the actual sounds of speech. Now we must realize that everything which may be expressed through the medium of these gestures,—and which is therefore in a certain sense the revelation of man himself, just as the spoken word is also a revelation of man himself,—we must realize that all this is based upon the possibilities of form and movement inherent in the human organism. For this reason we may choose yet another starting-point; we may, that is to say, take the nature of man himself and develop from this the various possibilities of form and movement. We may see what manner of movement can proceed out of the human organism; and then, carrying this further, we may eventually discover how the individual movement can take on the character of the visible sound.

To-day, in the first place, we will take our start from the actual being of man, and we will endeavour to discover the forms and movements which may arise in this way. Then, proceeding somewhat further, we shall ask ourselves: Which sound is to be regarded as related to this or that particular movement?

For this purpose I shall need quite a number of eurythmists, and I will therefore ask them to come on to the stage.

Will you place yourselves in a circle, in such a way as to have equal distances between each point.

I. Raise both arms upwards, the palms of the hands turned outwards and all the fingers widely spread.

II. Hold the right arm closely to the body, the left hand being lightly supported against the side.

III.   Both arms stretched forwards, the one laid over the other.

IV.   The arms held to the sides, the left arm at some distance from the body.

V.   One foot placed forwards, the left hand grasping the right elbow.

VI.   Close the left hand into a fist and place it against the forehead; with the other hand, which is held more in a forward direction make this gesture.

VII.   Both hands forwards, the left hand below, the right above.

VIII.   Stand with the weight on the left foot, holding the right foot slightly raised, the right hand upwards in a vertical position, and the left arm bent somewhat sideways.

IX.   Bend the head forwards and downwards, touching the chin with the right hand, and allowing the left hand to hang at the side.

X.   Clasp the right arm over the head, covering the larynx with the left hand.

XI.   Place the feet so that they are turned inwards and cross the arms.

XII.   Left arm placed against the breast, the right arm against the back.

Here you see a series of gestures.   These gestures in their totality represent the entire human being,—the human being split up, as it were, into twelve separate elements, but still the entire human being.

You might also imagine these gestures being carried out by a single person, one after the other.   If you picture them being made one after the other by the same person, you would see still more clearly how in this way, when one individual makes all the movements, the whole being of man is revealed and expressed with a quite remarkable force and clarity.

Let us now pass through these several aspects of the human being.   We will begin here (gesture IV, page 160).

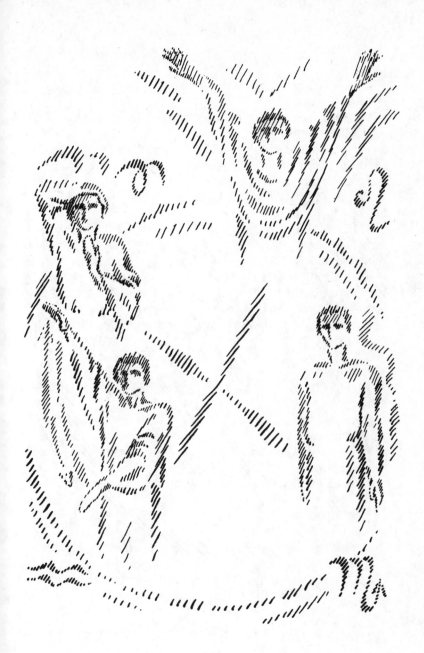

159

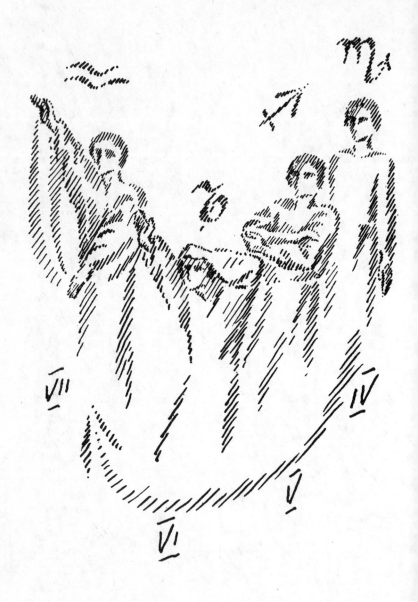

160

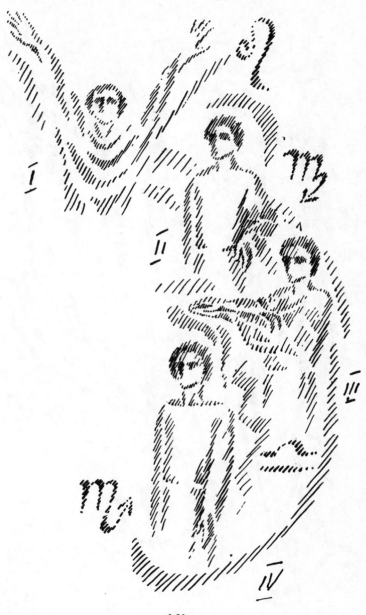

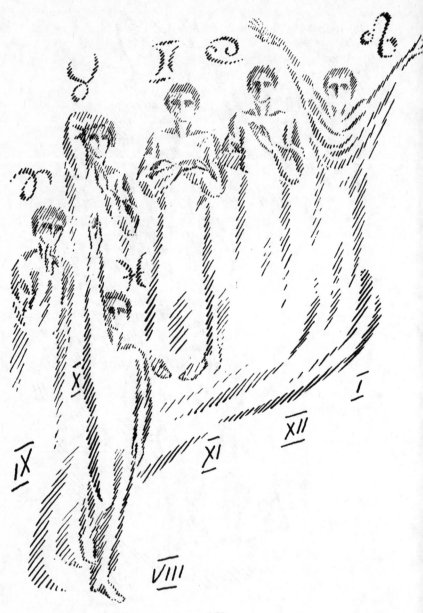

162

Try to imagine that we here have represented that element in the human being which we call the intellect, the mind. We must realize that this gesture is the expression of the understanding, the intellect.

Now let us look at this gesture (I):
From this gesture there streams out with a sunny radiance, that element which may be described as *enthusiasm*, which has its source in the breast. Thus we may say: gesture IV —the head: gesture I—the breast, enthusiasm.

Now let us pass to this point (gesture X).
Here the head is enfolded by the right arm, while the left hand covers the larynx. In this gesture we have represented that part of the human being which is the expression of the will,—(the Word is silenced).—We have man as the representative of the will, of all that can lead to action, to deed. Thus we may say: *the limb system, will, deed.*

Fundamentally speaking we now really have before us the threefold organism of human nature: understanding, feeling, will.

Then we still have that gesture which synthesizes all these elements in itself. You can see how here, in this gesture, there is the striving after balance (gesture VII).
A state of balance is sought between these various aspects. One may imagine that the arms move in this way (with an upward and downward movement), and that by this means one is endeavouring to experience this state of balance. Here we feel the whole human being, seeking to obtain equilibrium; it is the representation of the human being who finds *the perfect balance between his three forces,—thinking, feeling and will.* I will only write ' the human being in a state of balance '. You must take these descriptions which I am writing here as matters of the greatest significance.

Now we will go one stage further; when you pass over from the thinking human being to the human being as he seeks for equilibrium you have, lying between these two aspects, that element which follows after thought, which is the consequence of thinking. Where does thinking lead us?

163

To *resolve*. Thus gesture V is the resolve, the thought which wishes to transfer itself into reality. Resolve (see diagram V).

Now we reach this point (gesture VI).

We see from the very nature of this gesture that something exceedingly significant lies here. This gesture (IV) represents thought. Thought may be very clever, but it does not necessarily enter into reality; it does not necessarily reach the point of resolve. Here we have thought; but thought may always miscarry when it comes to a question of external matters. At this point (gesture VI) thought struggles with the conditions of the outer world: *the bringing of thought into connection with the external world* (*Auseinandersetzung des Gedankens mit der Welt*). This connection of thought with the outer world must actually become part of the complete human being; for the man who has reached a state of balance can, as he goes his way through the world, only bring his deeds to fulfilment when he has first entered into a relationship with the outer world.

And now, starting from the understanding, we will take the other direction. What really happens before one formulates a thought? Something must lead over to the state of understanding. Before a thought is actually formulated we have the state of hypothesis; we have a weighing, as it were, of the pros and cons of the matter. Thus here, in this gesture (gesture III), you see *the weighing process in its relation to thought*.

But how does this weighing, balancing process come about? In this connection we must make an accurate study of gesture II. What lies behind this gesture? You will remember that we take as our starting-point, feeling, enthusiasm (gesture I). This is a ' burning enthusiasm ' (the enthusiasm which we lack so greatly in our Society, but which at least is represented here). Now, passing from gesture I to gesture III, before we reach that quiet feeling of weighing or balancing, a reasonable soberness must first make its appearance (see diagram). Gesture II—*Soberness*.

You will be able to feel this quite easily if you enter into the gesture correctly and without prejudice.

164

We have, then, that enthusiasm which has its seat in the breast (gesture I). Now we come to this point (gesture XII).

Here we have not yet reached enthusiasm, rather, let us say, enthusiasm does not on this side pass over into a weighing, thoughtful process; it passes over into action, into the expression of will. On the path from enthusiasm to will, we find the first stage to be *initiative*, the going out of oneself, the impulse towards action. Enthusiasm burns with a fire which cannot endure. But when an action is to be accomplished there must be initiative, there must be the impulse towards action. Here then (gesture XII), we see *the impulse towards action*.

Now we must pass still further; let us observe the next stage. Here the whole human being is filled with the conviction that he will succeed in accomplishing the action (gesture XI).

We can almost see Napoleon before us. Special attention, too, must here be paid to the dexterity of the legs and feet; the eurythmist must not stand as in the other positions, but with a firm hold on the ground. You will notice that admirals on board ship always stand in this way. (And let me here advise you, when you are on a ship, always to walk in this way; then you will not so easily feel the motion of the vessel, nor so easily become sea-sick.) This, then, is not merely initiative, but it is the *capacity for action*. Here we have already reached the capacity for action.

And now, with gesture X we have the *action itself*.

Then we go one stage further. When the action has been accomplished, what has been brought about by its means in the world outside man? We see the human being living in the world. He observes what has been brought about through his action. It is no longer a question of the action only. The human being has already passed beyond this; he can observe it; action has already become event,—an event which has been brought about by his action, by his deed. Thus in gesture IX we have *the event*.

And now we pass on to gesture VIII.

In this gesture you can see that the event has made its

impression upon the human being. He has caused something to happen and this happening has left its impression upon him; it has become destiny. Thus we may say—*Event has become destiny.*

In this circle, then, we have the human being divided up into his component elements. We can picture this human being as containing within himself twelve elements and we can also discover the twelve corresponding gestures.

And now I need seven more eurythmists. Let us start here in the centre: Stretch out the arms, the right arm forwards and the left arm backwards; and now you must move both arms simultaneously in a circular direction. (You need, however, only actually make this gesture when all the others have been told what to do.)

With this first gesture which I have described we have no longer merely the gesture which is held, but one which is in movement. And when we take this gesture, this movement, we find that it is the expression of the human being *in his entirety.*

Now the second: left arm backwards, right arm forwards; you must move the left arm in a circle, the right arm remaining quiescent.

Here we have shown you the second movement. It is the expression for all the loving, sacrificing qualities in the human being. Thus: *the human being in his aspect of loving sacrifice.*

Now comes the third movement: right arm forwards, left arm backwards, the right arm moving in a circle. This is the extreme opposite of the preceding movement. It is the antithesis of the loving, sacrificing qualities. This is the *aspect of egoism.*

The fourth: stretch out the arms in front of you, with the lower arms crossed one above the other. This gesture is in the sphere of the spiritual; for this reason it may remain quiescent. Here we have everything in the human being which is creative; it is the *capacity for creation.*

Now we come to the fifth: you must hold the arms forwards with the fingers drawn inwards, and the movement is

166

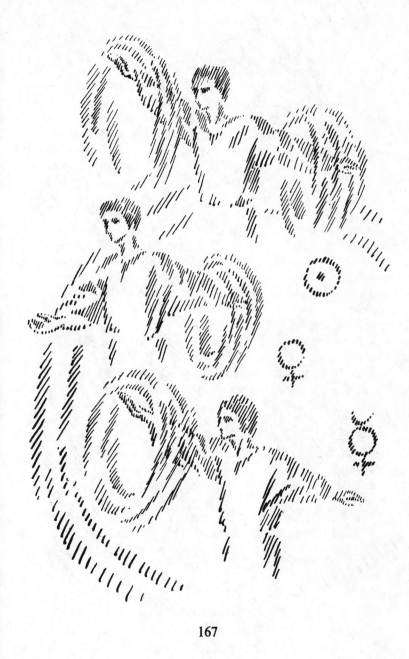

167

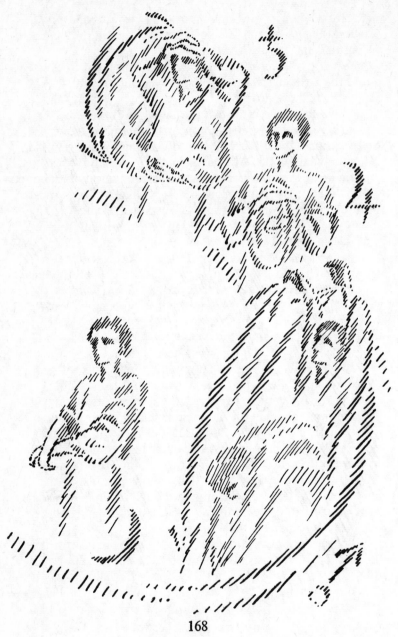

made by means of a rocking of the body, upwards and downwards. This represents the aggressive quality in the human being, thus the *aggressive element*.

The sixth: you must hold the left arm still (bent inwards) while the right makes a circular movement around it. In this way we show clearly that we are not now expressing the aggressive element but the *activity arising out of wisdom*.

And now we have the last movement: Here the hands are placed against the forehead, the one somewhat over the other; now allow them to move smoothly up and down,— and again, up and down. Make this gesture, this movement. Here we have the expression, of everything which is most profound, the contemplative, meditative element. The human being is here turned in upon himself; I will describe it as a *deep contemplation* (Tiefsinn).

Thus we have formed a large circle and also a small circle. In the outer and larger circle we have the twelve outer gestures which are static, which express form; here in the inner circle we have seven figures which express movement,— with one exception, that is to say. This gesture expresses a different aspect, namely movement which is brought to quiescence.

Now you will soon see what a harmonious effect is produced when all these postures and gestures are combined: those in the inner circle carry out the movements belonging to them, while those in the outer circle take up their postures.

We must, however, go still further: those in the inner circle make their movements; the outer figures move slowly in a circle from left to right, always holding their postures. During the whole time the others also must make their movements. Here, you see, it is as though the human being were observing the world from all sides, and bringing all his faculties and capacities into movement.

Will you once again take up your postures and form the outer circle? I must just mention that in eurythmy the direction from left to right is really reversed (that is to say it is taken from the point of view of the audience); this also applies to the direction from right to left. The outer circle moves at a moderate pace from left to right; those in the inner circle, still making their gestures, move round somewhat more rapidly. Thus the inner circle dances round at a rapid pace, the outer circle dances round more slowly. Now add all the movements and gestures. See what a harmonious effect is produced! This is one possibility. Here we have a first attempt at drawing forth from the organism its inherent possibilities of movement and gesture; and we can do this when at the same time we bear in mind the human being in his entirety. And we can indeed see how, in the future, further possibilities of form and movement will gradually be able to develop from out of this element.

In very truth the human being has not grown up simply from those forces known and recognized by present day science. He has grown up out of the whole cosmos and his nature may only be understood when the whole cosmos is taken into consideration.

When we have taken all that we have just seen and really observe it closely, then we may say that we have before us the human being divided up into all his different faculties, into the various qualities and forces of his being.

But, in the outer world, the human being is always divided up into the various members of his being. This is to be seen in the animals. The human being bears within him all the faculties of the principal animals. These are gathered together in him, synthesized and raised to a higher level.

Thus we have in the first place the four main animal types. Here we have enthusiasm, the breast element—*Leo*, the lion. The lion has as its dominant characteristic what we have here in this its corresponding geture (I).

Further: Here (X) is that element which is manifested in the outer world in everything standing under the sign of external action, under the sign of the will: *Taurus*, the bull.

Then here (VII), you have that which seeks to blend in the human being as a whole all the elements of experience, of action: you saw this in the way the movement was shown. Here we have that which welds together all the separated qualities, just as the etheric body welds together all the different members of the physical body. At one time the etheric man was also called the ' Water Man'. Here one really ought to write: The Etheric Man. According to ancient designation, however, this is also the ' Water Man ', —so here I may justifiably write: *Aquarius, the Water Man.* You now know that this signifies the etheric man.

Then we have the fascinating quality of cleverness, of brains, that which creates an impression (IV). And it is just here that tradition has brought about a gross error. In reality this has to do with all that is connected with the innermost organization of the head. So that I ought really to write: *the eagle.* This confusion between the eagle and the scorpion seems, however, only to have arisen in comparatively recent times. Here then, we must picture the eagle (see diagram). But everywhere to-day we shall find this sign designated as Scorpio. (I do not necessarily mean to imply that people have gradually learned to regard the understanding as something which stings them!)

Now we have here the four main characteristics of the human being. The others lie in the intervening spaces; enthusiasm does not immediately pass over into action; something lies between. At this point, we have initiative (XII). This impulse which leads us over from enthusiasm to activity, which takes us out of ourselves, is incorporated in the feeling system, in that part of the human being which is enclosed by the ribs. In the ancient language of physiology this part of the organism was designated as ' the crab'. Here also, then, I may call this point: *Cancer, the crab.* In the zoology of earlier times the word ' crab ' did not merely signify that animal which we to-day call the crab; it signified all those animals possessing a specially strongly developed rib-organization. This is what was originally meant by the word ' crab '. Everything which had a special development of the ribs was ' a crab '.

Now when the human being wishes to pass over into the sphere of action he must be able to move properly; he must bring both sides of his organism into a properly balanced movement. Thus the element of left and right in the

171

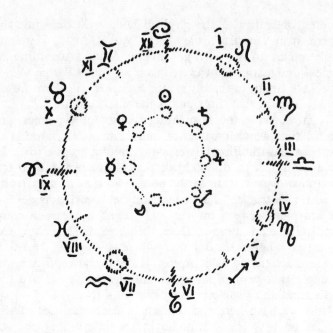

human being must be brought into action in a harmonious manner. Here we must observe that type of animal which is so organized that it has continually to bring the left and right sides of its organism into a synthetic and harmonious movement. Some animals, when walking or running, have to do this to a very marked degree: *Gemini, the twins* (XI).

As I said, from here we pass on to the action, and from the action to the event. When we examine this transition from the action to the event we find, in the animal kingdom,

CONSTELLATIONS OF THE ZODIAC		PLANETS
♈ = Aries = Ram	♎ = Libra = Scales	☉ = Sun
♉ = Taurus = Bull	♏ = Scorpio = Scorpion	☽ = Moon
♊ = Gemini = Twins	♐ = Sagittarius = Archer	☿ = Mercury
♋ = Cancer = Crab	♑ = Capricorn = Goat	♀ = Venus
♌ = Leo = Lion	♒ = Aquarius = Waterman	♂ = Mars
♍ = Virgo = Virgin	♓ = Pisces = Fishes	♃ = Jupiter
		♄ = Saturn

that it is best symbolized by those animals having curved horns. This brings us to the event: *Aries, the ram* (IX). Naturally, I should have to speak at considerable length if I wished fully to justify this statement.

Then we go further and reach the point where the human being is merged in the external world, where he gives himself up to the external world; we come to the point where his action becomes destiny. Here the human being lives in the moral element as the fish lives in water. As the fish is merged in the water in which it swims, almost becoming one with it, so does the human being live with his destiny in a moral outer world. Thus: *Pisces, the fish* (VIII).

Now I have already said that one must find a gradual transition from enthusiasm to quiet thought. We find this transition when the burning enthusiasm becomes sobered. The cooling element, that element which has not yet caught fire, when embodied in the animal kingdom, was called in ancient times: *Virgo* (II).

And after this soberness comes the quiet, weighing process, the balancing: *Libra, the balances.* Those animals which seem to consider everything were, in the dim past, designated as the balances.

Now we pass from IV to VII, from Scorpio, or more properly the Eagle, to Aquarius, to the etheric man. First we have the resolve, where thought determines to make itself felt in the outer world. It is easy to see why certain animals which dart from place to place from a certain nervousness of disposition, as for instance, certain woodland animals, it is easy to see why in ancient times such animals were named 'Archers', This is something different from what was later supposed; it is simply a characteristic of certain animals: *Sagittarius, the archer* (V) (see diagram). (To-day, even, I believe that in certain dialects the expression ' Schütze ' (archers) is used for those wretched little insects which dart about in the kitchen regions.)

And now we come to the bringing of thought into relationship with the world. At this stage, where one butts at everything,—where one has not yet achieved the blending of all the human qualities nor reached as yet the sphere of destiny,—at this stage we have the goat. Thus here I must write (VI): *Capricorn, the goat.* Man in his entirety is summed up in the circle of the Zodiac. But all this must be regarded as expressing human qualities and faculties, and these human qualities again make their appearance in the postures we have been studying.

Now in the inner circle we have had the expression of the human being as a whole: *Sun.* Next we passed over to the human being in his aspect of loving sacrifice: *Venus*; then to the more egotistical aspect: *Mercury*; to the creative, productive aspect: *Moon*; to the aggressive aspect: *Mars;* and then to the aspect of wisdom in the human being, that which radiates wisdom: *Jupiter.* And finally we have that which passes over into a certain melancholy, into an inner contemplation, into a profound inwardness: *Saturn.*

As we enter the sphere which reveals the human being to us in the way I have just described, we pass over from the postures which are held to the gestures which are in movement. And if we now wish to synthesize all this, to gather it together into a single whole, we can do so in the way I have shown you, by bringing the circle into movement. By so doing we externalize all that which together makes up the complete human being, that is to say, the synthesis of all the animal qualities, the animal characteristics.

A certain experiment is given in the ' Colour Teaching ' of Goethe: here one paints a disc in sections according to the seven colours,—red, orange, yellow, green, blue, violet, etc., then one brings the whole thing into movement, whirling it ever faster and faster until the whole impression is grey. The physicists assert: white,—it is however, not white, but grey. The separate colours can no longer be distinguished; everything appears as grey.

Now if the eurythmists had moved with such rapidity that the separate gestures were no more to be seen, but all were whirled together into a whole, then you would have seen something of extraordinary interest: the picture of the human being expressed through his own movements.

Here (in the inner planetary circle) you have all those qualities in the human being, which tend outwards, those possibilities of inner activity whereby the animal nature is gradually led over into the human. Thus, in the outer circle we have: *all the animals as man;* and here, in the inner circle we have: *a synthesis of the animal qualities transmuted into the human by means of the sevenfold planetary influence.*

And now I must ask you (the details I shall give you next time) to bear in mind the sounds,: *a, e, i, o, u, ei, au*—seven vowels. When we take the consonants really according to their innermost nature, grouping those letters together which are somewhat similar in sound, we get the twelve consonants. Thus we have twelve consonants and seven vowels. We arrive at the nineteen possibilities of sound when we see the consonantal element in the Zodiac, and the vowel element in the moving circle of the planets. This is the language of the heavens; whenever a planet stands between two signs of the Zodiac, in reality a vowel is standing between two consonants. The constellations arising through the motions of the planets are indeed a heavenly utterance, which sounds forth with infinite variety. And that which is here uttered is the being of man. Small wonder, then, that in the possibilities of gesture and movement the cosmos itself is brought to expression.

Such thoughts as these enable us to realize that in eurythmy we are really reviving the temple dancing of the ancient Mysteries, the reflection of the dance of the stars, the reflection of the utterances of the gods in heaven to human beings below upon the earth. It is only necessary by means of spiritual perception, to find once again in our age the possibility of discovering the inner meaning of the gestures in question.

To-day, then, we have discovered nineteen gestures; twelve static, and seven permeated with movement,—of which latter one is quiescent only because rest is the antithesis of movement. (In the Moon we have movement annulled by its very velocity.) Thus we have learned to know these gestures, and I have also been able to indicate how they lead over into the realm of sound. Here we have taken the human being as our starting point and have travelled the opposite path. Previously we started from the sounds; now we take our start from the possibilities of movement and follow this path till it leads to man, to a visible language, to the sounds themselves.

LECTURE 11

HOW ONE MAY ENTER INTO THE NATURE OF GESTURE AND FORM

Dornach, 8th July 1924

We shall now see how many of the difficulties with which we are faced in eurythmy are bound to arise if we do not work out of a deep and inward understanding of the gestures and movements as we learned to understand them yesterday. These difficulties present themselves when, for example, it is necessary to pass over from one consonant to another, or from one vowel to another; and you will have seen, from what has already been said, that as far as the spiritual element of language is concerned, what lies *between* the sounds is of paramount importance, just as in music that which is truly musical lies between the tones. The tones are the physical, as it were, the material element; the spiritual element of the music lies in the inner movement leading from one tone to the next.

In just the same way the spiritual essence of language is to be found in the *transition* from sound to sound. If, therefore, I am conscious of the existence of spirit in matter and on the other hand, am conscious that the sound as such is a physical, material means of expression, it will not be difficult for me to perceive that the spiritual element must necessarily lie in the transition from sound to sound. Yesterday we learned to know the spiritual significance, the spiritual reality underlying certain movements and postures. To-day we must try gradually to link up all that we learned yesterday with what we already know as the eurythmic formation of the sounds.

With this in view, we will begin as follows: First of all, I must ask those eurythmists who represented the Zodiac to take up the same position on the stage as they had

177

yesterday . . . and now we must add those who represented the planets. You know already from the previous lecture which of the animals in the Zodiacal circle each one of you represents, so that now I can ask you to note carefully what follows. We shall connect each of the signs of the Zodiac with a different consonant:

Aries: *v*

Taurus: *r*

These are really half vowel sounds, and should be thought of as vowels into which there enters a consonantal element. (Both are related to the vowel sound *a*).

Gemini: *h*

Cancer: *f* (in the German language *v* also)

Sagittarius: *g*

Capricorn   *l*

Aquarius: *m*

Pisces: *n*

Leo: *t* (Tao)

Virgo: *b*

Libra: *ts*

Scorpio: *z*

(It is essential, my dear friends, to take careful note of these correspondences).

Now we will take the inner planetary circle:—

Sun: *au*

Venus: *a*

Mercury: *i*

Moon: *ei*

Mars: *e*

Jupiter: *o*

Saturn: *u*

At this point I must ask each of you to take up your own position,—that is to say, each one of you must make the movement or gesture that you made yesterday. Now you must pass over from this movement to the corresponding sound, and from this sound return once more to your original position or movement.

In this way you get a gesture corresponding to the sound,

178

both preceding and following the sound itself; and it is from these gestures that you should seek to discover the transition leading from one sound to the next.

You will, of course, have to work out all this in detail later on, so that you do not lay undue emphasis on what lies between the sounds. To-day we have in the first place to see what can be drawn out of the constellation we have formed already, and which we now have standing before us. You each of you know your own sound, and must make it whenever it occurs. In this way the whole poem will arise out of a combination of 12 plus 7, and we shall see how a poem can be interpreted in eurythmy by making use of such a constellation. As a preliminary you must each make your own gesture or movement, and continue to make it while I begin to read the poem quite slowly. As the sounds follow one another you will each make your own particular sound as it occurs, passing into the sound from your previous movement, and returning to this again. (But you must all be as alert as terriers, because it is from out of the whole complex of sounds that the poem takes its shape.)

> Edel sei der Mensch
> Hilfreich und gut!
> Denn das allein
> Unterscheidet ihn
> Von allen Wesen,
> Die wir kennen.
>
> Heil den unbekannten
> Höhern Wesen,
> Die wir ahnen!
> Ihnen gleiche der Mensch;
> Sein Beispiel lehr' uns
> Jene glauben.

Now I shall continue to read the poem, and you will make the same movements you made yesterday,—movements which correspond to the zodiacal and planetary circles. At

179

the same time, while still holding the gestures, you will move round in a circle, each of you making your own sound as it occurs in the text. You will see that the effect is now much more beautiful:

Denn unfühlend
Ist die Natur:
Es leuchtet die Sonne
Über Bös' und Gute,
Und dem Verbrecher
Glänzen, wie dem Besten,
Der Mond und die Sterne.

Wind und Ströme,
Donner und Hagel
Rauschen ihren Weg
Und ergreifen
Vorüber eilend
Einen um den andern.

Auch so das Glück
Tappt unter die Menge,
Fasst bald des Knaben
Lockige Unschuld,
Bald auch den kahlen
Schuldigen Scheitel.

If you are careful to keep at exactly the right distance from one another, you will see how, by this means, by allowing the whole thing to develop out of a reality, out of the living movement of the circle and out of the spiritual gestures, each separate sound stands out against a background suitable to it, a background which embues it with a new spirituality.

What I have said in this connection is of the very greatest importance for those of you who have already learned the elements of eurythmy, and are far enough advanced to be able for instance to express in eurythmy such a poem as Goethe's 'Zauberlehrling'. This marks a quite definite stage in one's eurythmic development, and is, up to a point, a stage which may be regarded as complete in itself. But once having reached this stage it becomes necessary to work very intensively along the lines I have just indicated. For, by practising the gestures that you were shown yesterday, and by studying the way in which these gestures may be made to lead over into the individual sounds, an unusual, and at the same time most necessary flexibility will be brought into the fashioning of the sounds themselves.

See how beautiful it is when the eurythmist representing Capricorn frames her sound in such a way that, before and after the sound, this gesture makes its appearance. The sound, the letter, must be drawn forth from the gesture, and must be allowed to sink back into the gesture once more. In this way you obtain gestures which provide a frame for the sounds. In other words: a sound is correctly expressed in eurythmy only when,—well, shall we say at any rate, to some extent,—it is consciously made to grow out of this gesture, and to return to it again. It is, of course, obvious that these gestures can only be touched upon in passing.

You will also gain very much,—not as yet with regard to public performance, about which I shall speak later,—but for the actual learning of eurythmy, when you introduce these things into solos, duets, trios, etc. Let us take the case of a single individual, the eurythmist who represents Capricorn, for instance, and let us suppose that this eurythmist were asked to express a poem by means of consonants only, leaving out the vowel sounds. She would then have to choose the shortest possible way of getting to the place of the particular consonant in question, forming it only when actually reaching the spot. Then, passing on her way from this consonant to the following one she would have to make the gesture corresponding to the latter,—and so on, throughout the poem. These things are of the very greatest importance. By such means eurythmy can gradually be led over into the very nature of man's being, for the gestures are of such a kind that they are actually based upon the being of

181

man. Thus we gain the possibility of building up the whole form, the eurythmic form of a poem in such a way, that it expresses not merely the inner judgment of the individual performer, but in addition to this the living relationship between one eurythmist and another, when several are taking part, and a living relationship with space.

Now to-day you will naturally not be in a position to do more than carry out the particular movement, the particular sound each one of you has been given. At this point, however, we will for once permit ourselves to stand, not facing the audience in the usual way, but turned towards the centre of the circle, so that you can all watch the eurythmist who is making the consonants, each in its appropriate place. This eurythmist, after making a particular consonant,— for the moment we will leave the vowels on one side,— moves towards the place of the next consonant, and makes the movement expressing this towards the eurythmist representing it in the circle. . . .   You see how well it is going already, and how beautiful it looks.

The twelve eurythmists forming the outer circle have, therefore, to pay due attention to their own sounds. The first sound that occurs must be made by the eurythmist to whom the particular sound belongs; then the one who is running the form must be on the look out for the next consonant, and must move towards the eurythmist representing it. The latter must likewise be ready, and must make the consonant also. Thus both will make the *same* consonant face to face. You will see that in this way we get a very beautiful movement.

At a later stage the same exercise must be practised without the circle actually being formed. Then one eurythmist does the whole thing alone, as though surrounded by a phantom circle, and seeing in imagination each movement being carried out by a phantom eurythmist.

I will now read a short poem, and you will express it in the way I have indicated. Everybody must remain standing with the exception of Frl. S. . . . whom we will ask to undertake the moving part.

Ach—(now begin to move) ihr Götter! grosse
Götter (the *r* is here similar to *a*)

> In dem weiten Himmel droben!
> Gäbet ihr uns auf der Erde
> Festen Sinn und guten Mut:
> O, wir liessen euch, ihr Guten,
> Euren weiten Himmel droben!

In this way it will immediately become clear to you that the
forms which one makes, need in no wise be arbitrary, but
should always be built up on a sound and reasonable basis.
Nothing obvious or trivial should be allowed to enter into a
form. If, for instance, the word " Bauch " (stomach)
should occur in a poem, we should be going to work in quite
the wrong way were we to try and express this word by
means of a realistically shaped form. What we have to do
is to base our forms on language as such; we have to make
use of the forms lying hidden in the sounds and in the
spiritual gestures which we studied together yesterday.

And now we will see how beautiful it looks when we
express the same poem by means of the vowel sounds.
Frl. H. . . . will you take the principal part this time? The
others will join in with the vowels.

You know the relative position of the letters towards which
you have to move.

> Ach, ihr Götter! grosse Götter

Be careful to make no intermediary movement, but stand
still when no new vowel sound occurs. When the same
vowel comes twice running one should remain standing
quite quietly on the particular spot one has reached in the
form. In this way a very beautiful effect is obtained.

> Ach, ihr Götter! grosse Götter
> In dem weitem Himmel droben!
> Gäbet ihr uns auf der Erde

Just think what a splendid exercise you can make out of these few lines; they provide you with an example in which, having arrived at a certain spot with a vowel sound, you must stand quite still when it is repeated.

You can, however, only experience such an exercise in the right way, if you have developed a true feeling for all that lives in speech. I will take these first three lines as an illustration of my meaning. I cannot say that I will recite these lines; I cannot say that I will declaim them; but I will *intone* them in two different ways, so that you can see what really lies in speech, and what it is absolutely necessary for the eurythmist to feel if the content of a poem is to come to expression.

a i ö e o e ö e

i e ei e i e o e

ä e i u au e e e

You must realize how entirely different the feeling is when we have: der Erde—*e e e*, compared with the feeling that arises when one vowel sound follows another. If you practice such exercises you will become very sensitive to these things.

Something similar is to be found in the consonants also, and it is upon this that the beauty of the poem largely depends. It is, moreover, fundamentally true that one has in no way mastered speech if one does not prepare a poem in some such way as this: To begin with, the vowels should be made to ring out while the consonants are barely indicated, and then the vowels should be allowed to fall into the background while the consonants resound in their turn. Just imagine the mood, the character you get by taking the consonants:

ch hr g tt r gr ss g tt r

n d m w t n h mm l dr bn

g b t hr ns f d r rd

fst n s nn nd g t n m t

184

In this way you have entered into the feeling of the vowels and consonants, one after the other. And it is this which the eurythmist must make a point of practising; then the body will become supple; it will actually be what it must become if it is to be used as an instrument. You must have a certain reverence for eurythmy if you wish to be eurythmists. This reverence must become conviction. If you are actually to imitate all the movements made by your larynx when you say even a moderately complicated sentence, then indeed you have much to learn. You have learned it already in your pre-earthly life.

In earthly existence we have some slight repetition of this in the response made by the larynx to the sounds heard in the environment, for the larynx imitates such sounds. In the spiritual world, however, knowledge of this kind is never acquired intellectualistically, but is of such a nature that it is intimately connected with feeling. By means, therefore, of exercises such as those we have been practising here, the feeling life is intensified and stimulated.

The point is not so much that we should immediately think of *performing* this Dance of the Planets (Planetentanz); for then, having decided upon this dance, for which one requires 12 plus 7 people,—thus 19 people in all,—we are liable to be told by those for whom the performances are to be given: 'You must please bring only seven eurythmists (including dressers), for we cannot possibly afford more.' So there you are; what is one to do? If the matter is rightly understood the point will be not so much the actual performing of such a Dance of the Planets, but rather the making of one's own all that has been given in these two lectures dealing with the transition from the spiritual gestures to the gestures expressing the sounds. If you do this you will have done much towards making your bodies supple, and you will develop a fine and delicate feeling for what is essential in eurythmy.

In this course of lectures we wish not only to go once more over the old ground, but also to consider everything which is likely to further the progress of eurythmy.

Now this progress is often hindered by the belief frequently held that it is not necessary to study eurythmy in order to be able to do it. Certain people have even gone so far as to wish to be teachers of eurythmy after having watched eurythmy performances for a matter of two or three weeks. Imagine how ridiculous such pretensions would be considered with regard to music or painting! We must gain sufficient insight into these things to know that eurythmy is something which makes man, in accordance with the possibilities of his organism, into an instrument, a means of expression. This, however, can only be achieved if those things are also practised which are not necessarily intended to be shown, but which, nevertheless, help to develop that suppleness of movement essential to performance. Consider for a moment all that is done by those specializing in other arts. You have probably all heard of the famous Liszt piano,—very likely other composers have made use of it also,—a piano having keys but no strings. Liszt practised on this piano; he always had it with him, and practised on it constantly. He naturally did not do this in order to make music, but in order to acquire technical dexterity. His neighbours heard nothing of it; thus it is good for other people also when one practises in this way! The neighbours are not disturbed the whole night long; one can practise throughout the night without disturbing a soul. It is only there for the purpose of bringing about organic flexibility.

What we have been studying in these two lectures is absolutely fundamental to eurythmy in that it brings into the organism an eurythmic technique of movement and posture.

After this digression we will go back to the last lines of the poem:

' Festen Sinn und guten Mut: '

Think of all we have here, of all that we absorb into ourselves with these words: *Und gu* (you must remain quietly in *u*) *ten* (you return to the previous place); *Mut*. The gradual finding of one's way into the movement which one feels to be natural when passing from one vowel to another or which one feels to be natural when the same vowel occurs more than once in succession, this it is which creates the right mood and impression.

> ' O, wir liessen euch ihr Guten
> Euren weiten Himmel droben! '

By this means it is possible to experience the vowels and consonants in their juxtaposition. In this connection I must expressly point out that it is not a question here of absolute position; I might just as well have asked the eurythmist representing *t* (Leo) to stand somewhere else, in which case the others would then have grouped themselves accordingly. . . . In any case, you come to different places when the whole circle moves. It is not a question of absolute position, but of the relative position each has to the other. On reflection you will see how great are the possibilities of form to be obtained in this way. These possibilities arise when one takes one's start from a particular spot: for instance, we might begin a poem with *t* . . . and obtaining thus a definite starting point, something to hold on to, we can proceed to make the form accordingly, for we know in what direction we now have to move.

Thus the main thing is to understand that by studying the content of the lectures given yesterday and to-day it is possible to find one's way into the essential nature of gesture and form.

LECTURE 12

Dornach, 9th July 1924

We will now pass on to certain things which have arisen
out of the fundamental nature of eurythmy, things which
are, up to a point at least, known to you already; and we
will then establish a connecting link between what I have
been speaking about and what you already know.

The first thing I wish to speak about is this: We have seen
how what might be described as certain moral impulses,
which we have brought before our souls in the numbers
twelve and seven, find their expression in human gesture, in
gesture which is either static or permeated with movement;
and we have seen how thought, in the sense of eurythmy,
is altogether possible on the strength of experiences and
judgments of the human soul, which shed themselves into
the sounds of speech.

That which thus streams out from the human soul in
gesture and movement can, however, also work back upon
the human being as a whole. And this is the basis of the
curative action of eurythmy, which may be effective, not
only in the sphere of the moral, psychic life, but also in
the physiological, physical life.

The curative action of eurythmy upon the moral and
psychic life will be especially apparent when certain eurythmic principles and facts are applied during the years of
childhood.

Now starting from this standpoint,—from the way in
which on the one hand form and movement arise from a
certain mood or attitude of soul and then re-act back once

more,—I should like to speak further of certain things which have already been dealt with, so that in these next days we may gain a somewhat wider outlook and make another step forward in the development of speech eurythmy.

You will all know the exercise which is specially adapted to bring one person into contact with another: the so-called *I and You exercise*. You stand in a square; on account of the audience, however, the two at the back must be a little closer together. And now you can do this exercise in the following way: *I and you, you and I, I and you, you and I— are we*. Here you have a real ' we ', the final joining together in the ' we ' (circle). The two who face each other in a diagonal direction are intended as the ' I ' and ' you '. As you approach each other you must clearly express the fact that you wish to belong one to the other and that the others also wish to belong to the circle; the diagonal line expresses the transition from the ' I ' to the ' you ', *you and I* . . . then retrace the line (this can be done many times in succession) . . . then the whole is consciously brought together: *are we*. If the exercise is to be repeated one can return to the starting places with *you and I, you and I*.

Such an exercise can be worked out in the most varied ways, taking as one's basis such aspects of the soul life as we have learned to know during the last few days.

Let us now suppose, Frl. V. . . . that you are the Eagle, you Frl. St. . . . Aquarius, you Frl. S. . . . Taurus, and you Frl. H. . . . Leo. Now make the gestures. You take these gestures as the starting point and return to them when the whole exercise is completed.

You must realize what you have thus expressed. You have, by means of this exercise, expressed the fact that the human being contains these four animals within himself in their aspect of moral qualities, and that when he becomes conscious of his true self, he understands that the whole human race is contained within his own being—thus, as man he really comprises the ' we '. Begin with these gestures . . . follow with the exercise . . . then pass with a certain grace back to the first gestures. Here we have an example of how these things which we have just learned may be applied.

In this way the whole exercise is brought to a right conclusion. Preliminary gestures; *I and you, you and I, I and you, you and I, are we;* concluding gestures. You then have the right introduction and the right conclusion, and the whole thing stands, as it were, enclosed in a frame.

Now this exercise is most excellent in the teaching of eurythmy from an educational point of view. Indeed, when one has observed in a child the tendency towards jealousy and ambition—qualities which one wishes to eliminate—one must persuade such a child to do this exercise with special warmth and ardour. In the art of education it is, of course, obvious that one must never apply anything having the least trace of what might be called magic; for anything of the nature of magic would work with a powerful suggestive element. It would re-act on the unconscious life of the child. Such means can only be used in the case of children of weak mentality, of deficient children; it is only permissible in such cases. When, however, abnormal characteristics are present in the soul life of the child it is absolutely necessary to work directly into the psychic life,— though here, too, of course, one must avoid anything in the nature of actual suggestion or magic. Now what really happens when four children do this exercise? They hear the constant repetition: ' *I and you* '. This brings to their consciousness the element of belonging together, of comradeship, the element of relationship to other human beings, and this is further impressed upon them in the: ' *are we* '. The gestures accompanying the exercise simply express the fact that the child is learning to pay attention to what is being done, to what is inwardly working upon him. Thus there is not the least trace of suggestion. It can really be said that this dance is a remedy against jealousy and false ambition. It can only be used in the case of healthy children when it is carried out with full consciousness, quite without anything in the nature of suggestion or magic.

But now you will ask: How does the case stand with pathological children? With pathological children one has to reckon with a consciousness which is already dimmed and clouded. Then, to a certain extent, suggestion does come into play. For this reason, the moment one enters the sphere of the pathological in children, one must clearly realize that although this exercise may be applied with excellent results to children whose consciousness is dulled, it should never be used with children whose minds are over active.

It is such things as these which prove that everything in the domain of curative eurythmy must only be applied in close co-operation with a doctor and working under constant medical supervision; for as soon as we enter the domain of the pathological only a doctor is qualified to form an opinion.

Let us pass to another exercise or dance, which has arisen out of a definite attitude of soul. In order to give this exercise a name, we have called it the *Peace Dance*. And this Peace Dance serves the purpose of teaching one individual in conjunction with others how certain nuances of the soul life may find their expression in eurythmic forms.

Let us suppose that you make some sort of a triangle. Make it so that the form looks something like this:

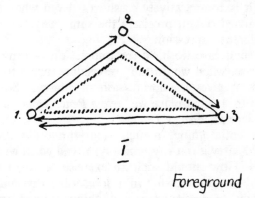

Foreground

Now one person can walk the lines of the triangle in this direction (arrow); or we can have three people, of whom the

191

first takes this line, the second this line and the third this line (see diagram).

When you look at this type of triangle and compare it with one of the following type:

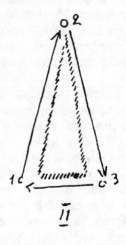

you have a considerable difference. In the first case one line is conspicuous on account of its length in comparison to the two other lines, and in the other case it is conspicuous because it is comparatively so short. Even when the exercise is carried out in precisely the same way, we receive a quite different impression.

In the first case we have the impression of peace; in the second case, when we do the exercise according to diagram II, the form gives the impression of energy. So that we may say: In the first place we have a *Peace Dance* and in the second place an *Energy Dance*.

The essential thing in such a eurythmic exercise is that we should carry it out rhythmically. And when we now ask ourselves: How should such an exercise be carried out?— we must bear in mind that in a descending rhythm we have what might be described as something ordered and under control, while in an ascending rhythm we have an element of striving, of will.

192

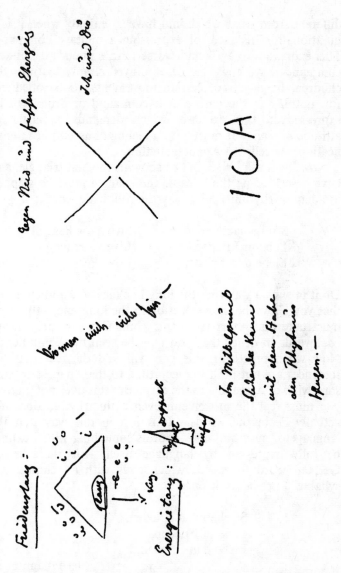

Now when we enter either into the mood of peace or into the mood of energy we have something of the nature of striving, of working towards some goal,—something quite

193

different from what we should have to employ when it is a question, for instance, of expressing a military command. This expression may sound worse than I intend; a military command may, however, be employed simply to train the children, by means of certain movements, to be obedient. But nothing in the nature of a command or order can be expressed in this exercise, which demands a particular attitude of soul. It must have a feeling of ascent, of intensification; it needs the Anapest rhythm.

Now I will ask Frl. S. . . . to show us the first triangle, as I have described it; the lines of the triangle must be stepped in Anapest rhythm while I say the following words:

Strebe nach Frieden,	(Strive for Peace,)
Lebe in Frieden,	(Live in Peace,)
Liebe den Frieden.	(Love Peace).

Do it in such a way that the long line faces the audience and that you show the intensification in the long line,—thus you must take your start from this point (1); you only move backwards in order that you may be seen by the audience. Now when practising this you will find the fact that the sentences are not built up according to the Anapest rhythm somewhat disagreeable to the ear. But this does not matter; you must feel the movement, even if this rhythm does not actually lie in the words. It is just in this way that the language of eurythmy may express something which cannot be fully expressed by language itself,—for there is no German word for peace which ends with an emphasized syllable. Let us try it once more:

> Strebe nach Frieden,
> Lebe in Frieden,
> Liebe den Frieden.

(see diagram I).

Show the Anapest very distinctly. The words are in the Dactyl rhythm, but in spite of this they must be stepped to the Anapest; the rhythm does not go with the words, nevertheless the dance must be done in the Anapest, without allowing oneself to be disturbed by the words. It would be better to use a text written in Anapest rhythm, otherwise there must be a certain disharmony, which is naturally disturbing to the ear.

Will you now do the next exercise. Here one must move, in Anapest rhythm, the triangle which has the short main line. Start once more from this point (1); try also to emphasize the form of the triangle by stepping the long side lines quickly, the short main line with a quite slow Anapest. This exercise may be called the Energy Dance.

These two exercises may, however, be carried out by a group. Let us now choose three people, who will first do the Peace Dance, taking their places in a triangle and each one moving one line only. This can naturally be done to a suitable text, which must be in the rhythm of the Anapest.

But this exercise can be done in yet another way. Triangles of similar shape, but small, may be formed in the four corners. Indeed this exercise may be carried out with any number of variations; but each variation will differ in its beauty. The best way perhaps, is for those standing at the point marked 1 to begin the form; they begin, and each one carries out a complete triangle,—but simultaneously. Eurythmy depends to a certain extent upon presence of mind. Each separate triangle must do a form similar to the triangle which previously took up the whole of the stage. Now all those standing at the back of the triangle, thus those whom I have placed in the corners, must do the *I and you* as the second part of the exercise: *I and you, you and I, I and you, you and I: are we.* Those who stand in the middle simply turn round. The triangle is thus built up in a different way. Those who now form the square must once more carry out the Peace Dance from their present places,— —the movement three times. When this is done smoothly and well it forms an exercise complete in itself.

From an educational point of view, as also from the point of view of curative education, this exercise, as we have just

195

done it, is of special value. One can make the group smaller using two or three triangles, but one can still carry the exercise out in a similar way. It is specially good to practise this exercise when one has, for instance, a class containing children of choleric temperament, children who will not be kept in order. Such children must be made to practise these exercises; and if this is done every day, or as often as there is a eurythmy class, for a period of two or three weeks, one will find that they have become more manageable. Thus children who are always hitting each other and rampaging about should be made to practise this exercise, and you will

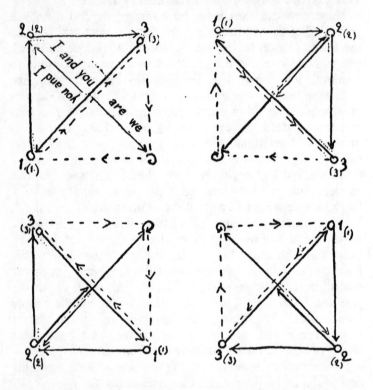

see that it has a remarkable power of soothing and quieting them.

Now we can do the Energy Dance in a similar way. Here again we must form our four triangles, but pointed triangles this time. Let us move the form of the triangles three times. Four eurythmists will now be standing in the corners (see diagram), and they must do the following exercise: Begin with the *u*, ' You and I '; with the ' I ' you are in the centre; now you have not the same gesture as you had for the ' you ' but you have a gesture which looks, as you stand together, as if you were going to attack one another. Go back once more from the ' I ' into the ' you ', and do this three times. Now you have reached a position from which we must go further. In the first place we do, as it were, the *I and you* exercise reversed, thus a *you and I* exercise: You and I, I

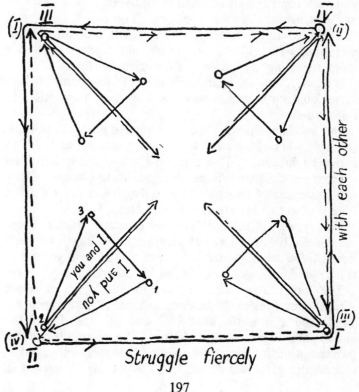

Struggle fiercely

and you, you and I, I and you, you and I, I and you—now you are standing at the back, and to continue the exercise you must run past each other crossing on the way (the four at the outer points changing places). Thus we go towards the centre; *You and I, I and you; you and I, I and you; you and I, I and you, struggle fiercely with each other, struggle fiercely with each other* (streiten heftig miteinander)! And now again the original exercise in the triangle three times repeated.

Do the whole exercise once more: the triangle three times, then the separating movement, then the triangle again.

In order to show you how such exercises may be multiplied and varied, we will do it as follows: move the triangle for the first time, for the second time, for the third time; now you must regard all those standing in the triangle as involved in the struggle. Thus do the form: You and I, I and you, you and I, I and you, struggle fiercely with each other, (thus everybody who is taking part); then make the triangles once more, repeating the form of the triangle three times.

It is, of course, comparatively easy to find poems of three verses built up in such a way that they may be practised to this form.

I should like to point out once more that it is quite possible to apply what you have just seen to education and also to curative education. This exercise has a specially beneficial effect upon children who are phlegmatic and sleepy. They will be stimulated by it; it will give them more inner vitality. That is what I had to say in this connection.

To-day we will take still another exercise, which is based more directly on the actual form. Out of the form itself you will feel what is intended. Frau B. . . . will you try to run a spiral form winding from within outwards.

The way you did this was perfectly right. You began with a quite noticeable movement, that is to say, with the hands laid against the heart . . . and you ended with the arms held in a backward direction. When you observe the movement of this form you will find that it is well suited to express the going out of oneself, the gaining of interest in

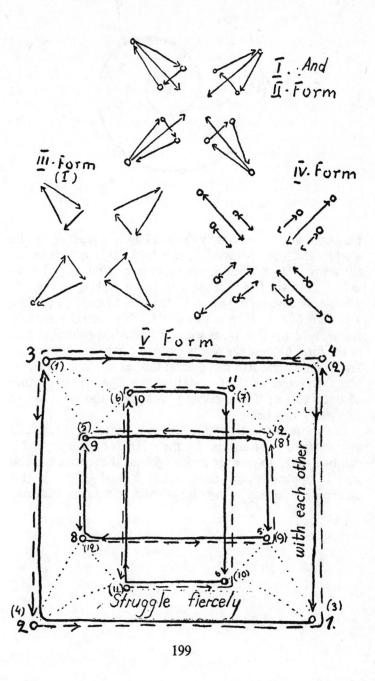

Ⅰ. And
Ⅱ. Form

Ⅲ. Form
(Ⅰ)

Ⅳ. Form

Ⅴ Form

Struggle fiercely

with each other

199

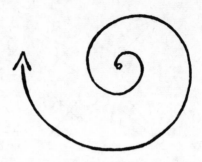

the outer world, and finally the yielding of oneself up to the world, which is expressed in the backwards movement of the arms. Do it once more, bearing in mind what I have said. You will feel that there is first a seeking in oneself, afterwards a becoming aware of the world outside, and then a yielding of oneself up to this world. Now run the reversed spiral; take the line from without inwards, in the first half of the form holding the hands more in a backward direction, and in the second half laid against the heart. You see this is just the reverse of the former line; it is a gathering together of one's forces; it is a coming back from the outer world into one's own being.

In curative education, this first spiral exercise is specially applicable to children who are the reverse of anaemic, and it can be applied to combat undue egoism; the second exercise may be applied where the ego-force is weak, and it is also an excellent remedy in the case of children who are anaemic.

LECTURE 13

Dornach, 10th July 1924

To-day we will continue to develop such forms as we spoke about yesterday. In this connection I should like to speak about those forms which may help to establish a certain relationship between a statement and its answering statement (Rede und Gegenrede). Yesterday I mentioned the spiral form and we saw how the evolving spiral gives the feeling of an outgoing of the human being into the world, and how the involving spiral gives the feeling of coming back into oneself. Now, however, let us bring these two forms into a relationship with each other. Move the forms to a clear Anapest rhythm; do it in the first place so that one form follows after the other. You can try it in this way: Frl. S. . . . will you take the spiral which goes from within outwards, and you, Frl. V. . . . the line which goes from without inwards; now reverse it, taking about six Anapests . . . it can be practised in this way.

In the case of dialogue,—a conversation from some play for instance in the form of question and answer,—it is good to move the spiral which winds from within outwards and which corresponds to the answer, in such a way that, when one reaches the last two Anapests, one simply takes two long, emphasized steps; it is as if one wished simply to have the long, emphasized beats. Do the exercise thus: Four Anapests, two long beats. In this way you get a form, the feeling of which corresponds to the nature of dialogue in a play, for example,—or indeed any dialogue which is to be expressed in eurythmy.

This form can also have a certain significance in curative education. I said yesterday that the one spiral form can be made use of in the handling of wild, unruly children, who are always fighting; while the other spiral may be used in handling children who are phlegmatic and who hardly come to the point of raising their own hands.

If you get individual children of such types to practise these forms you will have a certain amount of success. But if you form two groups—the one group of choleric, the other of phlegmatic children—and make both these groups run the spiral forms, and in such a way that the children must constantly look into each other's eyes, then they will mutually correct each other. If you employ this corrective action of the one type of child upon the other, these forms will prove to have a remarkably powerful effect.

Now we have in the course of the past years made use of a number of eurythmic exercises and forms, based on such

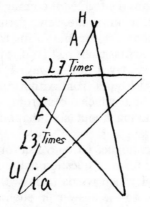

things as these. Frau. K. . . . will you do the form which we have for *Hallelujah*. One can, in the first place, do this to the pentagram form. You stand at the back point of the pentagram and use one line to do the ' Hallelujah '. Begin with the *H*, pass over into *a*, do the *l* seven times; pass on to the *e;* make the second *l* three times; then *u, i, a.* You must, however, continue to move the form. The second line of the form must be done in the same way. Thus, when carried out by one person alone, this exercise is repeated five times.

Now let us take five people; when each one does this same exercise we again have a complete 'Hallelujah'. Frau K.... you move the first line; Frl. S. . . . has the next, Frl. Sch. . . . the third, Frau Sch. . . . the following line and Frl. V. . . . has the last line.

You must all begin at the same time. And you must be careful to space out the line in such a way that, when the exercise is completed, you have all arrived on your own places.

In this way, out of the lines of the pentagram, you get a complicated and ever changing form. When this exercise is carefully practised the effect is very impressive and does actually convey the whole character of the word 'Hallelujah'.

It is, however, possible to find another variation of this exercise. Let one person stand here, the second there (see diagram) and there the third, fourth and fifth . . . now we must add a sixth and a seventh. Each one must move in this direction (see arrow).

A different impression is thus created. The form should be divided up as before. Those in the front must always stand in such a way that the back ones come into the intermediate spaces, and are, therefore, also visible. Let us try it: 1 to 2, 2 to 3, 3 to 4, 4 to 5, 5 to 6, 6 to 7 and 7 (in a curve backwards) to 1. (All at the same time.)

You will see that this produces a form of 'Hallelujah' which, on account of its measured tempo gives an impression of high exaltation.

Yet another variation can be brought about if each of you, on reaching your place (see following diagram), adds this line (the curve) to the form. (Here again all must move simultaneously.) The *two* lines of the form must now be accompanied by the same gestures as before. This way of doing the 'Hallelujah' necessarily entails a certain quickening of the pace. Such a form lends itself to many further variations.

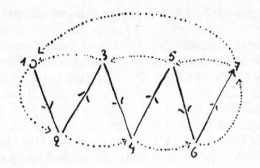

Let us for instance do it in this way: Frau S. . . . and Frl. Sch. . . . will you stand here, one on each side, while the others form the pentagram? Now, you Frl. Sch. . . . must make the movement for the Sun as we did it yesterday, continuing this while the others move the pentagram. At the same time, Frau S. . . . you must make the quiescent gesture for the Moon. Here we have a form for ' Hallelujah ' which again has its special colour.

Let us pass over from this form to our second form,—without the curved lines,—then we shall have a very exalted ' Hallelujah '. And in making this transition, let the Sun and Moon take their places as before.

At this point we can pass over to the last form of all, which again demands a somewhat quicker tempo. Thus the ' Hallelujah ' may be carried out in the most varied manner. In this way you get a form which will really have a profound effect upon the onlookers. Let us try it: *Hallelujah*.

This shows the possibility of making use of forms in such a way that they actually correspond to the most individual characteristics inherent in the matter in question.

Now let us vary the form of *Evoe* in a somewhat similar fashion. Frau P. . . . will you do it alone? With *E* take a step; with *v* stretch out one arm and with the other make a movement as though you were going to take hold of something; with *o* hold the arms to the sides and raise yourself up to a very erect position; with *e* step backwards. When you carry out these movements the form comes of itself.

Now let us see how this works out when done by three people. Here, when three take part, you can approach so closely together that each one lightly takes the hand of the other (with the *v*). The greater the number taking part in this exercise the more beautiful is the effect.

These are examples of definite forms which may be developed when, by entering into their inherent mood and feeling, and at the same time retaining throughout the true character of eurythmy, one is able to conjure up a certain mood of soul from out of the movements for the sounds.

It is also possible, by means of a single gesture arising directly out of a certain mood of soul,—as do the sounds in eurythmy,—to give adequate expression to some special feeling. Frl. S. . . . will you do the following: Dr. W. . . . will kindly stand here on the stage, while Frl. S. . . . looks at him; she must stand with the toe of the left foot touching the ground, and, while still looking at him, must make the movement for *S*; I think no one could mistake the fact that her dealings with him are ironical: the mood of *irony* is expressed absolutely naturally when this eurythmic movement is carried out in the right way.

And now, Frl. S. . . . will you make the following movements: first express an ironical perception of something, and then, with an inner effort of will make this mood of irony still more active. Thus we have the previous movement as the first stage; and now, putting the foot flat on the ground and still retaining the *S*-gesture, hold the chin awry and slant the eyes. Pass over from the first movement to the second: first *Irony*, then *delight in being a minx*.

There can be no doubt that we have here an adequate means of expression, one which is actually drawn out from the gestures themselves. You have seen how satisfying it is. I wanted to show by means of this example how these things must be felt and experienced.

In eurythmy the possibility of becoming truly artistic first arises when one has reached the point of finding each movement,—whether vowel, consonant, or any of the other movements we have had,—as inevitable as this most characteristic gesture for irony. From this very gesture you can learn how one can find one's way into all these things.

I want to show you another example of the metamorphosis of form. Those who took part on the stage yesterday in the interwoven *Peace Dance* and *I and You* exercise will remember how the four groups of three people were arranged; and I shall now ask those who were on the stage yesterday to come up again and take these same places. Let us do the following: instead of merely moving the form silently as yesterday, you will do the first form, the triangle, three times, accompanied by lines built up according to this pattern: Es keimen der Seele Wünsche,—then a second line to the second part of the form, and a third line to the third part of the form. We have now reached the point where yesterday we began the 'I and you'; but here again we shall have words which may be built up according to the pattern of 'I and you'. Thus we shall have a number of lines fashioned in this way. Then again, as an ending, we have another three lines, so that we once more come back to the *Peace Dance*:

> Es keimen der Seele Wünsche,
> Es wachsen des Willens Taten,
> Es reifen des Lebens Früchte.
> Ich fühle mein Schicksal, (approaching each other)
> Mein Schicksal findet mich, (going back)
> Ich fühle meinen Stern, (approaching)
> Mein Stern findet mich. (going back)
> Ich fühle meine Zeile, (approaching)
> Meine Ziele finden mich. (going back)
> Meine Seele und die Welt
> Sind eines nur.

Now come the last three lines corresponding to the Peace Dance:

Das Leben, es wird heller um mich,
Das Leben, es wird schwerer für mich.
Das Leben, es wird reicher in mir.

(The wishes of the soul are quickened,
The deeds of the will wax and grow,
The fruits of life are ripening.

I feel my fate,
My fate finds me.
I feel my star,
My star finds me.
I feel my aims,
My aims find me.
My soul and the world
Are one.

Life will be clearer round me,
Life will be heavier for me,
Life will be richer in me.)

In this way we have a relationship with the 'I and You',
etc. which is not merely schematic, not merely an abstract
form, but which, even if not perfect, is still absolutely
dependent upon the structure of the lines of the poem.   It is
an example of how these forms may be developed.   Do it
once more.   Now you will understand it better; you will
see that there really is a perfect adjustment between the lines
of the form and what is contained in the lines of the poem.

Here, at the same time, I have given you an example of
the intimate relationship existing between the language of
eurythmy and the language which we ordinarily use.

I have attempted,—it is naturally only a slight attempt and
intended merely as an illustration,—to answer the question:
How did poems arise in certain Mystery Centres where an
art of movement existed such as we are endeavouring to
renew in eurythmy?—In these Centres it was not the
language, the structure and form of language in a poem

which was considered in the first place, for a man of those early times had something within him which caused him first to experience the movement, the gesture with its accompanying form. And it was out of the form, out of the gesture, that the structure of the poem was sought. The eurythmic forms and gestures preceded the fashioning of the poem.

These things actually show the intimate relationship existing between eurhythmy and the earthly language. As eurythmists we must acquire a feeling for the fact that not every poem can be expressed in eurythmy. You see, at least 99 per cent of the poems which have gradually accumulated are far from artistic; at the outside we have the remaining 1 per cent. The history of literature could certainly not assume vast proportions if true poetry only were taken into consideration. For true poetry always contains eurythmy within it; it gives the impression that the poet who wrote it first carried out in his etheric body the eurythmic movements and gestures; it is as if he only possessed his physical body in order to translate the eurythmic gestures and movements into the language of sound. In no other way can a true poem arise.

Naturally this need not penetrate into the intellectual consciousness. Even in our present age there are true poets who dance, as it were, with their etheric bodies before they produce a poem; and in earlier times too such poets existed, as for instance Schiller in his really beautiful poems. I do not mean those poems of Schiller's which should also be set on one side, but those which are a real poetic achievement. With Goethe, too, in the case of most of his poems, one really feels the eurythmic gestures lying behind the words. Indeed quite a number of poets may be said to possess this quality, albeit unconsciously. It is present in them unconsciously.

Now the eurythmist must naturally be able to feel, from the way in which a poem works on his organism, whether it is suited to eurythmic expression; whether, that is to say, he can answer the question: Was the poet himself a eurythmist? Had he in himself that something which I wish to express in form and movement?—It is when one feels this to be the case that one can enter into a certain inner relationship with the poem which is to be expressed in eurythmy.

Of course all this must not be exaggerated, for in the realm of Anthroposophy we must never become fanatics; it is possible to carry such ideas too far. We need not, for instance, advocate that only such poems as arose out of the Mysteries should be done in eurythmy, or such poems as are fashioned, as it were, after the manner of the Mysteries. On the other hand one would not, I imagine, choose a poem by Wildenbruch. It is such things as these which must be felt by eurythmists, otherwise they will not be able to enter into the true nature of eurythmy.

From this you will perhaps have gained some understanding of the intimate relationship existing between eurythmy and language.—And now I will ask Frl. S. . . . to do the following in eurythmy:

> Mein Freund, kannst du es nicht lassen,
> Mir das Traurige immer wieder
> In die Seele zu rufen?

(My friend, canst thou not refrain from ceaselessly calling up sorrow in my soul?)

Do it as follows. Take, for instance, a simple wave-like line as your form, and, when you come to the words: ' Mein Freund, kannst du es nicht lassen ' . . . begin definitely to accelerate the tempo, letting this acceleration be really visible; move the second half: ' Mir das Traurige immer wieder in die Seele zu rufen,'—at a quite definitely quicker tempo. Do this once more. Now let us reverse the process in the following sentence:

> Was seh' ich: es ist der Morgensonne Glanz!
> (What do I see: it is the glow of the morning sun!)

After ' ich ' you must try to retard the quick tempo with

which you began. You have here (first example) the transition in tempo from slow to quick, and here (second example) the transition from quick to slow.

When it is a question of will or striving, as in the first sentence, in which there is the impulse to check something, where there is a certain element of will: ' I do not wish him to call this up incessantly before my soul '—then we have a transition from a slow to a quick tempo.

And when it is a question of the effect of an external happening, thus when,—as in the second sentence,—we are incited to observe something, when we have to do with perception, then we must pass over from a quick to a retarded tempo.

> Mein Freund, kannst du es nicht lassen,
> Mir das Traurige immer wieder   = Will
> In die Seele zu rufen?

Was seh' ich: es ist der Morgensonne Glanz!=Perception.

You will feel that these tempi really give the possibility of expressing in movement on the one hand, will and on the other hand perception or feeling. And you will have to analyse poems in order to discover whether it is more a question of expressing will, of resistance in the movement, warding off something, or whether it is a question of expressing a yielding up of oneself, something in the nature of reverence or devotion.

In addition to this one can, of course, make use of the gesture for devotion. The effect will then be intensified. For there are always more ways than one of expressing such things.

LECTURE 14

Dornach, 11th July 1924

Just as in speech itself an inner understanding for the structure of language makes it necessary to divide words, according to the train of thought, into nouns, adjectives, etc., so, in eurhythmy, also these things must be taken into consideration. It is, of course, obvious that all pedantry must here be laid aside, and that the teaching of eurythmy from the aspect which we shall be developing here to-day must never be allowed to degenerate into those methods too frequently employed in the teaching of grammar in schools. But the eurythmist must be fully conscious of the way in which each single word,—a noun, for instance,—must be treated; for these details have their place in the whole scheme of the structure of language, by means of which the human being is enabled to express himself through speech. It is necessary then to differentiate between words which express the characteristics of things, descriptive words, and words expressing activities. Such words as describe the characteristics of things may be expressed in eurythmy by checking the movement of the form. Just at the moment when one wishes to express an adjective in eurythmy one must pause in the form and make the gestures standing still; the gestures must be made during a quiet interval in the form. On the other hand, when we are expressing some soul-content, as we do in ordinary speech by means of a verb, the point is to accompany the gestures by a *decided movement* in the form. Thus, gestures accompanied by movement, gestures carried out by the human being in motion, may be said to be the expression of the verb.

Now, one can sub-divide that which is expressed by means

211

of the verb in this way; we may have the expression of something passive or of something active, or of something prolonged over a certain period of time. A transient activity, a transient passivity, or a prolonged activity, a prolonged passivity,—it is according to this that we can differentiate our eurythmic gestures. When we wish to express passivity, a passive relationship to something, the gestures must be made while the eurythmist moves in a forwards direction, not in a backwards direction. Everything which is inwardly connected with suffering, endurance, with a passive attitude, may be expressed by making the gestures to a forward-moving form; everything active may be expressed by making the gestures to a backward-movement in the form; while everything, either active or passive, which is of the nature of duration, may be expressed by making the gestures to a form which moves from side to side.

Thus we are able to express the verbal element in a way which enables the onlooker to perceive what actually lies in the nature of the verb.

We will now apply what has just been said to the working out of a short poem; we will try to bring out these three forms of inner experience as they come to expression in the verb. Let us, then, examine the verbs as they occur in this little poem:

Konnt' schlafen nicht (I could not sleep)

Sleep is something,—at least in the case of healthy people,—which has a certain duration; so here we must express something which lasts over a period of time (see diagram).

Konnt' träumen nicht (I could not dream).

Now it may be said of dreaming,—and we must always analyse a poem in this way before working it out in eurythmy,—it may be said of dreaming that this also is something involving duration, but here at the same time a slight passivity is indicated. We must try to combine the side-to-side

212

movement in the form with the forwards movement, not now going directly forwards, but in a diagonal line. You could express ' dreaming ' by this form (see page 215). The poem continues:

Konnt' schlafen nicht,	{I could not sleep,
Konnt' träumen nicht	I could not dream
Da hört' ich drauss'	I heard without
Wie das Eis zerbricht	How the ice was shattered.)

In ' heard ' we have another verb; ' heard ' is quite obviously passive, so the line must be forwards. ' How the ice was shattered '; we must bear in mind here that something is being said about the ice. Let us inquire: Is this the passive mood or the mood of duration?—If we enter into the feeling of this phrase we shall realize that we have to do with the mood of duration, but that there is also the indication of something *happening*, of something active. The shattering of the ice is the reverse of the purely passive mood; it may even be said to make an aggressive impression upon us. We say: ' shattered ' . . . this crackling of the breaking ice is continuous . . . and at the same time we must express the active mood by moving up to a point in a backwards direction.

Then we have a line without a verb; at least there is only an auxiliary verb and we will not consider this for the moment.

Es war, als ob aus der Ferne	(It was as if from afar
Es sich nahete	Something approached
Wehete, lüftete,	Wafted, floating aloft,
Und in den Lüften es	As if something in the air
Atmete, düftete.	Breathed, sending forth fragrance.)

To approach, to be wafted, to float,—all these verbs express duration, but they have at the same time something active about them. Here, then, we must express these verbs: ' to

213

waft ' ' to float ' by a line which goes backwards, and again
backwards; ' as if something in the air ' . . . here we have
no verb—' breathed, sending forth fragrance ' . . . must be
treated in the same way as ' wafted, floating aloft '.   We have
therefore, to move in a backwards direction, and then again
further back (see diagram).

Über die Felder her	(Over the meadows
Talherab, berghinauf,	Down the valley, up the mountain,
Wenn das der Frühling wär'	As though the spring were come
in vollem Lauf!	In full career!)

Now do the whole poem characterizing the different types of
verb:

Vorfrühling.	Early Spring.
Konnt' schlafen nicht,	(I could not sleep,
Konnt' träumen nicht,	I could not dream,
Da hört' ich drauss',	I heard without
Wie das Eis zerbricht.	How the ice was shattered
Es war, als ob aus der Ferne,	It was as if from afar,
Es sich nahete,	Something approached,
Wehete, lüftete,	Wafted, floating aloft,
Und in den Lüften es	As if something in the air
Atmete, düftete.	Breathed, sending forth fragrance.
Über die Felder her	Over the meadows
Talherab, berghinauf—	Down the valley, up the mountain
Wenn das der Frühling wär'	As though the Spring were come
In vollem Lauf!	In full career!)

We have then these different types of verb:*

---

* The reader should look at all diagrams as though facing a stage. Hence ↓ = a line
forwards.

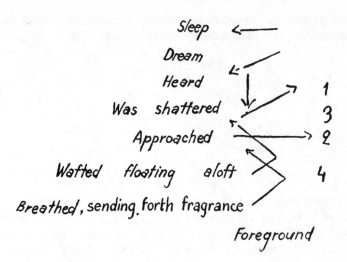

Now we must define the nouns. Here in the first place we have those nouns which describe such things as make an impression upon the senses, things which in ordinary life are termed concrete objects.

It is, of course, impossible to state definitely what is concrete and what abstract; this must be left to individual judgment. Hegel, for instance, protested against the usual conception of 'abstract' and 'concrete'. He declared that a washerwoman is something very abstract, whereas wisdom is absolutely concrete!

Everything depends upon whether one is able to conceive wisdom as something concrete and a washerwoman as an abstraction! Anyone who conceives wisdom as concrete will certainly feel that a washerwoman is merely existent in thought and quite without reality. A washerwoman has no real existence. The human being embodied within her exists, but, in her capacity of washerwoman, she is altogether unreal.

For this reason it is perhaps better to say: Objects which produce an impression upon the senses are described by words which must be expressed in the form by an angle backwards.   All objects producing an impression upon the senses correspond to a backward angle in the form.

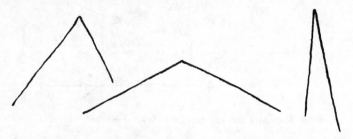

On the other hand that which in the ordinary sense of the word is termed abstract,—everything, that is to say, which makes no impression upon the physical senses but depends upon experiences of the soul, as for instance: wisdom, thought-power, genius, fantasy and countless other qualities, —everything of this nature must be expressed by means of a curved line in a forwards direction.

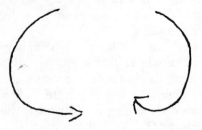

Thus the mental-contemplative element, as we may call it, is expressed in this way, and this gives us two separate forms corresponding with two classes of substantives.*

There is also another type of noun which expresses condition.   We might take as examples: whiteness, beauty, height.   In the case of these nouns of condition we reverse the form which we use for objects perceptible to the senses. We make the angle forwards.

* Dr. Steiner had previously given indications as to how words describing spiritual beings (God, Zeus, Dionysos, etc.) should be shown in the form.   Such words are expressed by a curved line backwards.

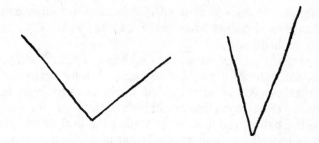

Then, further, we have words which express such things as are purely bound up with the soul-life. Here the curve line becomes more complicated.

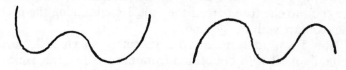

In this way we are able to show nouns expressing some mood of soul; yearning, suffering, pain, pity, good-will, and so on. By means of the angle forwards we express conditions which appear as attributes of external objects; while for everything dependent upon the inner soul-life we must use such a form as I have just described.

In this way you will discover movements capable of arousing in the onlookers shades of feeling and perception which will enable him to follow the inner laws which determine why a certain combination of sounds conveys a definite mood of soul, a distinct condition or sense-impression.

It is not necessary to move a separate form for each individual word; with the pronouns, as with the adjectives, the movements may be made standing still. Numerals also should be treated like adjectives; they need not, in so far as eurythmy is concerned, be differentiated from the ordinary adjective.

Interjections, on the other hand,—*Oh!* for instance, or *Ah!*—have a quite special significance, for it is by such words as these that beauty and grace may be brought into eurythmy. In the case of all interjections we must either introduce a bending movement of the body, or else a spring or little jump.

Now that I am speaking about a jump or spring I will take the opportunity of drawing your attention once again to the fact that everything of this kind which is introduced into eurythmy must be carried out in such a way that one jumps on to the ball of the foot, only putting the heel down later: there is something fundamentally harmful about any jump which brings one down on to the flat of the foot. Due attention must be paid to this; it has often been overlooked in spite of very definite warnings. In the case of every jump, including those which occur in tone-eurythmy, one must jump on to the fore part of the foot, later bringing the heel into contact with the ground.

Now I am going to make a statement which will most certainly meet with opposition from materialists, but which is, nevertheless, of the utmost importance for the whole sphere of eurythmy, for eurythmy in its artistic, educational and curative aspects. Every single movement from whichever aspect it is regarded, must be carried out with ' grace ' in the true sense of the word. And a eurythmy performance, or a lesson in eurythmy, which is not participated in by at least one of the ' graces ',—I do not, of course, mean this in a physical sense—cannot, my dear friends, be said to be justified. We must have the feeling: All eurythmy, educational as well as artistic, must be of such a nature that one of the Graces might look on without embarrassment.

This, of course, entails an energetic campaign against all lack of skill in eurythmy. And of all clumsy, awkward things this jumping on to the flat of the foot is the most awkward. As I have already said, every spring or jump must be on to the fore-part of the foot. When in education grace reigns in the sphere of eurythmy, the children actually grow in receptivity and perception in all directions. And teachers of eurythmy must make this increased power of receptivity and perception in the children the goal towards which they strive.

218

It is through grace alone that art finds its way into the realm of beauty. And in curative eurythmy,—this is the most difficult of all to believe, but it is nevertheless true, —one of the Graces must at least be hovering in the background. Even if not actually visible, she must be listening, and for this reason that every exercise of curative eurythmy not gracefully carried out tends to produce a stiffening and hardening effect in the etheric body, thus counteracting the desired results.

Frl. S. . . . will you now show us some eurythmy into which you must introduce graceful bending movements. You can be quite free to follow your own feeling; but, when I come to the third sentence, try in addition to introduce a graceful jump. With the first of these sentences the movements must be subtle and interesting. I am going to recite three examples; you can express each one by means of the vowel sounds, adding at the same time the movements which I have just indicated:

' The dog goes bow-wow '.

Introduce a bending movement which really represents the ' bow-wow '.

' The cat goes mi-auw! ' . . .

and now, with the third gesture, make three graceful little jumps, combining the last jump with some sort of bending movement:

' The cock goes cock-a-doodle-doo! '

In this way we get the interjections.

Further we have the prepositions. Some sort of acquaintance with these matters is, of course, essential. One must realize, for instance, that the prepositions express the relationship in which one thing stands to another. We have such words as: aus (out), ausser (outside), bei (with, among), entgegen (towards), mit (with), nach (after), nächst (next), von (of), zu (to), zuwider (contrary to),—all prepositions which, as we say, govern the dative; they are always followed by the dative, by the so-called third case. All prepositions must be expressed by a bending of the head and body in a sideways direction.

Here again, however, we must learn to differentiate. In the case of prepositions governing the dative the body must be bent, not sideways merely, but also slightly forwards, in a diagonal direction either to right or left; in the case of those governing the accusative the bending must be directly either to left or right; while in the case of those governing the genitive the movement must be sideways, and also slightly backwards.

In this way we get more variety. Let us now try to express the preposition in the following little poem. I shall ask Frau. P. . . . to express the preposition, when it occurs, by means of the corresponding movement.

' Was mag es bedeuten? '

This is a question. In this connection we spoke earlier of the spiral form and now we have an opportunity of applying it.

Was mag es bedeuten?
Mein Herz pocht so geschwind,
Die Glocken sie läuten
Im Morgenwind.   (Bending movement forwards and
                          sideways.)

You can, then, express prepositions in this way. On the other hand, a bending of the head *only* is the expression for conjunctions,—and, but, etc.—for those words whose function it is to connect other words and sentences.

To-day I want to speak of the way in which the structure of a poem may be shown by means of eurythmy forms. We must naturally try to make this course of lectures as comprehensive as possible, and with this in view I will now touch upon certain things which may help us to bring out the actual form of a poem, and to express this in eurythmy.

To begin with I will show you how one may treat a poem in which the same form of verse, the same inner structure of the verse, is constantly repeated.   We will suppose, for instance, that we have a verse of four lines, and we will see how such a four-lined verse can be worked out. . . .   There are, of course many other possibilities.   I do not mean to imply that

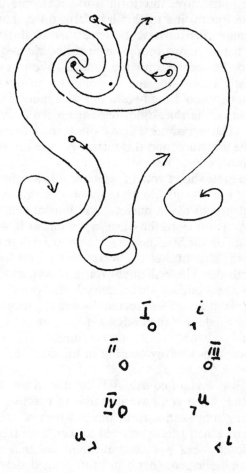

every verse of four lines must be built up in this way, but it can be so built up.

One eurythmist must stand here (1), and move the first form, trying to find his way into it for the first line of the verse. The second eurythmist who stands here, does this form, trying to find his way into the second line, and of course only moving when this second line is being recited. The third must stand here, and during the recitation of the third line must move this form (forwards); and the fourth moves the fourth line to this last form (foreground). But now we must also observe the structure of this verse and see how the rhymes occur; the first line rhymes with the third, and the second with the fourth. We can show this quite clearly by making the eurythmist who does the first line continue to hold the *i*-gesture. This must also be done in the case of the third line; here again the *i*-gesture must be held. The eurythmist doing the second line continues to hold the *u*-gesture; and this same *u*-gesture must be shown by the fourth eurythmist.

This example shows you, in principle, the way in which the forms and movements of eurythmy may be drawn out from the actual structure of a poem. Will four of you take these places,—you will learn the form in a moment by looking at the diagram on the blackboard,—and now I will read a poem in which the structure of the verse corresponds to the form just described. This will show you how you can find your way into the building up of eurythmic forms. For one must not build up a form merely by vague dreaming, or by indefinite, muddling methods; a form must be made to correspond to what is actually contained in the text itself; and this can be done by bearing in mind all that has been said.

You will at first, of course, only be able to move the form as such, but, when you have had time to practise, you must try to bring into such a form those details of grammatical structure to which I have referred to-day. All this can also be introduced,—but you need not think, when a movement forwards is indicated, that you must immediately take ten steps! The slightest indication is quite sufficient, and indeed the effect is most beautiful when these things are suggested only. To-day I will not impose too much upon you, but will ask you simply to run the form, not showing the additional grammatical details. To do this would be comparatively difficult, but it is nevertheless possible, with adequate practice. The poem runs thus:

Scheiden

Was mag es bedeuten?
Mein Herz pocht so geschwind.
Die Glocken, sie läuten
Im Morgenwind.

Was mag es bedeuten?
Mein Herz ist wund.
Die Glocken, sie läuten
Die Abschiedsstund.

Die Glocken, sie klagen.
Mein Herz tut mir weh,
Die Stund hat geschlagen
Ade, Ade.

Die Stund hat geschlagen.
Das Herz klopft so sehr.
Ich sitz in dem Wagen
Komm nimmermehr.

In this way then (see previous diagram), one can build up the form of a poem. To-morrow I shall speak even more exactly about the structure of poems; to-day I must just add the following:

It is only by repeatedly calling up a certain mood of soul that the eurythmist can gain the receptivity of feeling and perception necessary to expressive gesture. This delicate and fine perception can be awakened in the eurythmist by means of a meditation drawn out from the secret nature of the human organization. It can be attained when you enter, in deep and inward meditation, into what lies in the following words, not feeling them as words merely, as abstract concepts, but allowing their content to ripen within you. It is thus that you will be able to achieve all that I have just described.

I seek within me
The Strength of Creative Working,
The Power of Creative Life.
It tells me
The heavy weight of Earth
Through the Word of my feet,
It tells me
The forming power of the Air
Through the Singing of my hands,
It tells me
The strength of Heaven's Light
Through the Thinking of my Head,
So the World in Man
    Speaks, sings, thinks.

Ich suche im Innern
Der schaffenden Kräfte Wirken,
Der schaffenden Mächte Leben.
Es sagt mir
Der Erde Schweremacht
Durch meiner Füsse Wort,
Es sagt mir
Der Lüfte Formgewalt
Durch meiner Hände Singen,
Es sagt mir
Des Himmels Lichteskraft
Durch meines Hauptes Sinnen,
Wie die Welt im Menschen
    Spricht, singt, sinnt

When you have meditated upon such words as these, you will discover that you can say of yourselves: It is as though I

224

have awakened out of a cosmic sleep into the heavenly realm of eurythmy. If you stimulate this mood and feeling in your souls, you will be able to enter this realm as though awakening out of the darkness of night into the light of day.

LECTURE 15

IN EURYTHMY THE ENTIRE BODY MUST BECOME SOUL

Dornach, 12th July 1924

To-day we must bring this course of lectures to its conclusion. It has, naturally, only been possible to give certain guiding lines; much still remains unsaid and must be reserved for a future occasion. It seemed to me better to develop these guiding lines in a really fundamental way out of the nature of eurythmy itself, rather than to attempt a more encyclopedic survey of the whole domain of eurythmy.

It is of the greatest importance that each individual eurythmist should strengthen this power of creating the movements out of an inner activity, for it is in this way alone that a true understanding for eurythmy can be developed.

I shall deal first (my attention having been drawn to the matter) with the two sounds *g* and *v* (German *w*). Let us first take the *g*. In modern languages,—in modern European languages, at least,—this sound has not the same significance as it had in earlier times. For this reason we have not considered it until now. The sound *g*, when properly formed—*gg*—signifies an inner strengthening of the self, a strengthening of the soul-forces, a concentrating in itself of everything in the human being which *naturally* spreads outwards. It is therefore the sound of speech which, so to speak, holds our being together, in so far as the latter is a vessel for natural forces. This is the sound *g*.

Perhaps Frl. V. . . . will make the movement for *g*, in order that you may see how well the character of this gesture is adapted to show this inner strengthening and concentration. The warding off of everything external and the welding together of everything inward is expressed in the gesture for *g*.

Now we come to the remarkable sound *v*. We find this sound less frequently in the more ancient languages, in the

226

Oriental languages that is to say. It expresses a special need of the human soul. It is as if the human soul were not used to the shelter of a firmly-built structure, but felt compelled to wander. Instead of the firmly-built house which may be experienced in the *b*-sound, instead of this solid house, the soul feels the need of a tent, or of the shelter of the woods. In the *v*-sound there lies the feeling of what may be described as a moving shelter.

This is why one always feels, with the sound *v*, that one is, as it were, carrying a shelter which is constantly being set up anew. Everything of a wandering nature, where the essential element is movement, must be experienced in this sound. It is the surging of the waves which is expressed by a strongly formed *v;* when delicately formed it expresses the sparkling of the waters. This will help you to realize what must be felt in the sound *v*. Now it is a remarkable fact that, when using the sound *v* (German *w*), one quite naturally finds one-self repeating it. One feels compelled to repeat it several times in succession. Something seems amiss if one simply says: ' es wallet ' ; one wishes to say: ' es wallet und woget, es weht und windet, es wirkt und webt,' and so on. There is, in short, no sound which leads so naturally into the sphere of alliteration as this sound *v*. An alliteration can be made up with other sounds, but in no other way will it come about so naturally.

Perhaps Frl. S. . . . will demonstrate the sound *v*. You see how it demands a gesture filled with movement. *V* may thus be said to be that sound which permeates being with movement. Will you now show us, just going round in a circle without actually showing the structure of the alliteration,—we shall add this shortly,—an alliteration built up on the sound *v*. In this example there are also other alliterated sounds; but observe how slight an impression they make when compared to one built up on the *v*-sound (German *w*). Thus we have:

> Wehe nun,
> Waltender Gott,

227

Wehgeschick naht.
Ich wallete
der Sommer und Winter
Sechsig ausser Landes,
Wo man mich immer scharte

(now comes the other alliteration)

In die Schar der Schützen,
Doch vor keiner Burg
Man den Tod mir brachte.

Then we have a very marked alliteration, built up on *m;* you will feel this strongly, yet not so strongly as in the case of *v:*

Nun soll mein eigenes Kind
Mich mit dem Schwerte hauen,
Morden mich mit der Mordaxt!
Oder soll ich zum Mörder werden?

One cannot help feeling that every alliteration based upon the *v*-sound appears to come about quite as a matter of course, whereas all other alliterations, no matter what sound is repeated, have the effect of being drawn out from the *v*.

Alliteration is an essential and fundamental element in poetry, especially where the sound *v* is experienced in a living way. In this connection we must develop a two-fold feeling. In the first place there lies in the nature of alliteration,— that is to say, when the first letter of certain words is repeated, —something which takes us back into earlier stages of European culture. *Wilhelm Jordan* has attempted to revive alliteration, and has indeed succeeded in introducing it into his work with a certain strength and conviction. In modern German this element of alliteration appears somewhat out of place. A feeling for it, however, can always be recaptured if one has the gift of going back in imagination to an earlier epoch. The short poem which I have read to you is taken from the Song of Hildebrand. Hildebrand was long absent from his native country, and on his return journey he met his son Hadubrand with whom he came into conflict. It is the battle between these two which is related in this alliterative form,—a form which was at that time an instinctive and completely natural means of expression.

An alliteration may be shown in the following way: Let a number of eurythmists form a circle, and now,—because the very essence of alliteration is consonantal, although not invariably based upon the v-sound,—they must emphasize the alliterated consonants by stepping round this circle. The vowel sounds do not form part of the alliteration; for this reason they may be shown by another group of eurythmists who stand inside the circle, making the movements for the vowels.

I will ask several of you to show the alliteration in the poem I have just read. Will you take your places in the circle; and now three others must stand in the centre and show the vowels.

The alliteration will be particularly strongly emphasized if, whenever a new alliterated sound occurs, it is shown by a different eurythmist, the preceding eurythmist at the same time repeating the previous sound. Only those vowels which follow directly after the alliterated consonant should be shown by those in the outer circle. The other vowel-sounds must be done more as an accompaniment by those standing in the centre. In order to make the whole thing quite clear let us take this example and do it quite slowly, those in the outer circle moving to the alliteration:

*We*he nun,
*Wa*ltender Gott,
*We*hgeschick naht.
Ich *wa*llete
Der Sommer und *Wi*nter
Sechsig ausser Landes,
Wo man mich *scha*rte
In die *Scha*r der *Schü*tzen,
Doch vor keiner *Bu*rg

229

Man den Tod mir *bra*chte.
Nun soll mein eignes Kind
*Mi*ch mit dem Schwerte hauen,
*Mo*rden mich mit der *Mo*rdaxt!
Oder soll ich zum *Mö*rder werden?

The alliterated consonant and the vowel sound immediately following it must be carried round the circle from one eurythmist to the next.

This will show you how in fact movement, and also restraint may be brought into such a poem sheerly by means of alliteration.

We will now pass on to something else, something which will help us to make of the human organism a fitting instrument for the service of eurythmy. In this connection it is very necessary to gain an understanding of the difference in eurythmy between *walking* and *standing*. Standing still always signifies that one is the image, the picture of something. Walking, on the other hand, signifies that oneself will actually *be something*. When working out a poem in eurythmy you must be able to feel whether, at a certain point, it is a question of describing or indicating something or of representing the actual nature of something in a living way. It is according to this that one must decide whether to stand still (a lessening of the movement tends already in this direction), or whether to pass over into movement. We shall find that we have less occasion to stand still than to move, for there lies in the very nature of poetry the tendency to express something living, something which *is*, not merely that which signifies something. Here it is well that we should know how the human body is related to the whole cosmos. The feet of man correspond to the earth, for in their very structure they are suited to the earth, Where we have to do with gravity, with the weight of the earth,—and this feeling of the weight of the earth is present in nearly all forms of human suffering,—we must endeavour to express this in eurythmy by a graceful use of the feet and legs.

230

The hands and arms reveal the life of the soul. This soul-element is the most essential part of what may be brought to expression in eurythmy, and this is why in eurythmy the movements of the arms and hands play such an important part. Here already we pass over into the realm of the spiritual, for it is in the transition from one sound to the next that we find the best means of expressing that which is spiritual. In language the spiritual element finds expression in the mood of *irony*, for instance, or roguishness, in everything that is to say which emanates from the human spirit (aus dem menschlichen Spiritus), from man himself in that he is a spiritual being, gifted with intelligence in the best sense of the word. Such things must be indicated by means of the head, for the head is the instrument of the spirit.

We must become conscious of such things; then we shall be able to express them in the right way. It is specially important to be able to use the head in the most varied manner according to the possibilities of its organization.

Frl. S. . . . will you turn your head towards the right. The turning of the head towards the right may always be taken to signify: ' I will '; naturally I do not mean these two words merely, but everything which contains the feeling: ' I will.'

On the other hand, when you turn your head towards the left it signifies: ' I feel.' Thus, everything in a poem where the mood of ' I feel ' is dominant we must turn the head towards the left.

Now bend the head towards the right. This bending movement of the head (forwards towards the right) signifies: ' I will not.' Bend it in the same way towards the left and it signifies: ' I do not feel this, I do not understand it or realize it.'——

And now bend the head forwards, straight forwards. You will see how natural this movement is if you do the following: Frau Sch. . . . will you stand facing Frl. S. . . . in profile, and do these movements. We must suppose that Frau Sch. . . . says: ' It is the gods who inspire the human heart with willing service.' Frl. S. . . . gives an eurythmic answer: ' You are too clever for me; I do not understand you.' She shows

231

this by means of the aforesaid gesture, carried out clearly and definitely. You will find numberless opportunities of applying this movement. It signifies a sinking into oneself when faced with something which one is not able to understand.

Then, further, so that we may have at least one example, I must point out that the twelve gestures related to the Zodiac and the seven gestures related to the moving planetary circle may be made use of in a variety of ways. Quite apart, for instance, from what was said yesterday with regard to rhyming we must learn to understand such an exercise as the following:

Frl. S. . . . and Frl. V. . . . will you demonstrate what I am now going to describe. Frl. S. . . . will you make the gesture for Leo, and you, Frl. V. . . . the gesture for Aquarius; now, as I read this little poem, try to show it in eurythmy. In the case of the emphasized rhymes, the rhymes which fall on an accented beat, you, Frl. S. . . . must make the gesture for Leo. With the unemphasized rhymes, thus those which do not fall on the accented but on the unaccented beat, you, Frl. V. . . . must make the gesture of Aquarius. Make the movements standing still, choosing perhaps the vowel sounds, and only making the zodiacal gestures at the end of the lines so that we may really see their effect when they follow immediately after the rhyme.

Es rauschst das Bächlein über Gestein. . . .

(You, Frl. V. . . . must hold the sound)

Ein Weidenbaum drüber gebogen,
Drauf sitzt des Müllers Büblein klein,
Im Schosse ein kleines Zitherlein,
Die Füsschen bespült von den Wogen.
Es kommt ein Mann des Wegs zu gehn,
Er bleibt so still, so schweigsam stehn
Sieht zu dem sinnigen Knaben;
Hatt' auch ein Büblein klein,
War auch so still und auch so fein.
Das liegt nun draussen begraben.

You see how the rhyme may be emphasized in this way by means of the zodiacal gestures. I am drawing your attention to such things so that you may be able to work out similar exercises for yourselves, thus gaining assurance and certainty in the development of eurythmic gestures.

I will now ask a number of eurythmists to come forward and make various movements as I explain them: Number one must place the feet together, stretching the arms out so that they lie in a horizontal direction, on a level with the shoulders.

Number two must stand with the feet slightly apart, holding out the arms in such a way that the hands about correspond with the level of the larynx:

Now for number three: stand with your feet somewhat further apart, and hold the arms in such a way that, if a line were drawn from hand to hand, it would pass just below the heart.

Number four: stand with the feet still further apart, quite wide, holding the arms right up above the head. The hands must be held in such a way that they could be connected with the feet by means of a straight line.

Number five: stand with the feet in a similar position to number three, and now hold the arms in such a way that a line drawn from hand to hand would pass at the level of the top of the head.

Here (in the case of Number two) the line passes across the larynx; here (Number one) the line is quite horizontal; here (Number four) it is high up above the head; and here (Number five) it is just at head-level. Continue to hold all these gestures.

Number six: you must stand with the legs close together, with the arms held upwards in an absolutely vertical line:

To these gestures we must add the following words:

Ich denke die Rede	I
Ich rede	II
Ich habe geredet	III
Ich suche mich im Geiste	IV
(meinen geistigen Ursprung)	

233

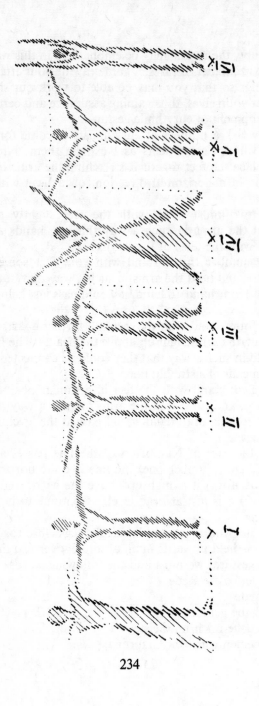

234

Ich fühle mich in mir   V
Ich bin auf dem geistigen Wege   VI
Ich bin auf dem Weg zum Geiste (zu mir).

I think speech
I speak
I have spoken
I seek for myself in the Spirit
   (my spiritual origin)
I feel myself within myself
I am on the spiritual path
I am on the way to the Spirit (to myself).

Approximately in this way. And now you must try to pass from one position to the next. Frl. V. . . . will you do this? Place yourself in front of each one in turn, and, as you take up each position, you must feel impelled to express the words that are said by means of the gesture being carried out by the eurythmist standing behind you. As Number one, you have to begin:

Ich denke die Rede.

Passing on take up your place in front of Number two:

Ich rede
Ich habe geredet
Ich suche mich im Geiste
Ich fühle mich im mir
Ich bin auf dem Geistwege.

In this way we get the whole series of gestures.

Ich denke die Rede
Ich rede
Ich habe geredet
Ich suche mich im Geiste
Ich fühle mich in mir
Ich bin auf dem Wege zum Geiste (zur mir).

235

If, when teaching eurythmy to adults, a beginning is made with this very exercise, it will certainly help them to find their way into eurythmy easily and well.

These gestures, when carried out in this way one after the other, form an exercise which may be classed among those having a harmonizing and curative effect. Thus, when anyone is so much disturbed in his soul-life that this disturbance works itself out into his physical body, manifesting itself in all sorts of digestive troubles, then this exercise, taken in such a case as a curative exercise, may always be given with the greatest benefit.

And finally, my dear friends, I must once again impress upon your hearts the fact that really good eurythmy can only be achieved when there is the determination always to make a thorough and careful preparatory analysis, of anything which is to be interpreted by means of eurythmy. Every poem must be studied in the first place with a view to discovering which are the most fundamental sounds. If in a poem expressing the feeling of wonder, the wonder experienced by the poet, we find many *a* sounds, then we may be quite sure that this poem is well suited to eurythmy, for it is the sound *a* which expresses wonder. The poet himself has felt that *a* is specially related to the mood of wonder. And the eurythmist will be able to intensify the effect by laying stress on the movement corresponding to the sound *a*. In eurythmy it is even more important to concentrate on the sounds contained in a poem than on the actual sense-content of the words. For the sense-content is the prose element. The more a poem depends upon its sense-content, so much the less is it a poem; and the more the sound-content is brought out, the more a poem is dependent on sound, the nearer it approaches to true poetry.

As a eurythmist, then, one should not take one's start from the prose-content, but should enter so deeply into the nature of the sounds as to be able to say: When many *a*-sounds occur in a poem it is obvious that it is a poem based upon the mood of wonder and must be so expressed. This shows us the attitude we must have towards language as such. Further we must seek in poetry for those characteristics of language which we have already mentioned here,— what is concrete, for instance, what abstract, and other details of this kind. This means that one must first enter into the nature of a poem and study it according to *the structure and formation of its language*, only later trying to express it in eurythmy.

In eurythmy there is still another thing to bear in mind, and that is the way in which, in the eurythmy figures, I have tried to portray *Movement, Feeling and Character*.* This is another field of study for eurythmists. The movement must be felt *as movement*, and is depicted as such in the figures. As a eurythmist one lives in movement. We must, however,—more especially when a veil is floating around us, but also when we are not actually wearing one,— picture this veil as expressing the aura (see Eurythmy Figures). It is only when one bears this in mind that one can bring the necessary grace and beauty into the movements. Let us look at the eurythmy figure for *l*. The *l*-sound itself lies in the movement; but that which can be added to the *l* as feeling, is shown by the fact that here, in the region of the arms, the aura is quite wide, becoming narrower as it hangs down. You must imagine that your arms reveal your feeling by means of the floating aura of the veil. The dress which here appears somewhat wider at the bottom must be studied in a similar way. This is how one must picture oneself. As a eurythmist, one should always feel oneself attired in dress and floating veil as I have indicated here in the figure.

Character also is of the greatest importance. When stretching out the arms one should actually feel that here (see figure) the muscles are stretched and taut. Everywhere where *character* is indicated by means of its corresponding colour there must be a tension of the muscles. This must also be shown by the eurythmist. And here again, for example, (see figure) you must use the legs in such a way that you really experience this muscular tension. The

* See page 274. The Eurythmy Figures.

237

eurythmy figures are intended to show such things and have been designed accordingly.

When you have in this way made a study of each separate sound, your whole organism will be so sensitive to sound that you will feel: This whole poem is built up upon the mood of *l*, let us say, or upon the mood of *b;* and it will then be possible for you to create your interpretation of a poem out of the sounds themselves.

All these things must be very carefully borne in mind when it is a question of teaching eurythmy. In educational eurythmy it is naturally important to introduce such movements of the body as can work with moral benefit upon the soul-life, and serve to further the development of intellect and feeling.

In artistic eurythmy the essential thing is that the soul should gain the power of working through the medium of the body. Thus the movements of eurythmy, these gestures as they are shaped and formed, must be felt to be absolutely natural, indeed inevitable. One must feel that they could not be otherwise, that it is only by means of these very gestures that certain moods or artistic concepts can be expressed.

Yet another thing must be borne in mind, and that is the fact that the learning of eurythmy entails an actual transformation of the human organism. Any performance which reveals the slightest trace of struggle between body and soul must be looked upon as unfinished and imperfect. In a eurythmy performance the whole body must have become soul.

A programme is sometimes given—as you yourselves know—which has been prepared with unbelievable industry and is then shown for the first time. One can enjoy such a programme, where everything is fresh and spontaneous, where there is still a struggle with the form-running, and where on occasion the arms are not moved but thrown about, appearing so heavy as to be liable at any moment to fall to the ground. There is spontaneity in all this and it gives us a certain pleasure.

238

Then the time comes when the programme is taken on tour and given perhaps in some ' two dozen ' towns. (As a matter of fact, I believe this has never actually happened, but it might well happen.) The programme is, as I said, performed in about two dozen towns and the eurythmists return. Then,—because Frau Dr. Steiner has had no time to prepare a new programme,—this old programme, which we saw some six weeks ago in all its youthful spontaneity, is presented again. Now the pleasure is of a very different kind. Everything has become easy and fluent. One notices, too, that the eurythmists, because they have visited new towns and learned to know fresh conditions, are stimulated by the outer world and have gained a certain inner enthusiasm. All this has had its effect on the movements and they have become effortless and free. The performance is now sheer delight, and one can only exclaim: ' Oh, if this programme could be performed fifty times more, how beautiful it would be then! '

We must have an understanding for these things. Every artist whose work is bound up with the stage knows the truth of what I have just said. A good actor would never think that he has mastered a role before he had played it some fifty times. With the fifty-first performance he might perhaps think that he could play the part, for then everything would have become second nature. We, too, must acquire this attitude of mind, my dear friends. We must develop such a love for anything which is to be shown in a performance that we simply cannot put it aside. Indeed no one but the onlooker may be permitted to find an often repeated item dull or tedious! It is in the sphere of art above all, that it is important to realize this; one must come back to a thing again and again. In a place where I once happened to be staying, I had the opportunity of seeing a play repeated fifty times. I went every evening to see this same play and allowed it to work upon me. By the fifth evening I did perhaps have a certain feeling of boredom, but by the fifty-first evening I was not in the least bored. Even though the performance, in a small provincial theatre, was very mediocre, so much could be learned from its very imperfection that this experience,—peculiar though it was,— could be of life-long benefit. As a matter of fact, I did not like the play in question; as a play it did not interest me at all. (It was Sudermann's *Ehre*.) I could not stand the play; nevertheless, I saw it performed fifty times by a somewhat mediocre cast. My aim was to enter into all the details unconsciously, thus experiencing it purely with the astral body. I wished to take it right out of the realm of conscious perception and simply to live with it.

People must learn,—and now, when I am speaking about eurythmy, I will take the opportunity of mentioning it,— people must learn the value of rhythm, even in more complicated matters. We say the Lord's Prayer not fifty times only, but countless times, and we never find it tedious. Notice is seldom paid to the fact that such things are connected with experiences of the human organism, experiences which are apparently more or less immaterial and to which our Karma leads us at one time or another.

With this, my dear friends, we must bring this course of lectures to a close. From the way I have developed the subject, you will have realized that my first aim has been to show you that it is out of the feelings, out of the soul-life, that eurythmy must proceed. Eurythmic technique must be won out of a love for eurythmy, for in truth, everything must proceed out of love.

How much I myself love eurythmy, my dear friends, I have told you recently in the ' News Sheet '.* I said then how earnestly I wish that the great devotion demanded of all those actively engaged in the work of eurythmy,— work which was begun by Frau Dr. Steiner, begun by our eurythmy artists here in Dornach and which has gradually won wider recognition and esteem,—how earnestly I wish that all this may be rightly appreciated; for it cannot be too highly prized in Anthroposophical circles. It is my hope that this course of lectures may have contributed something towards the furthernace of eurythmy in this respect, in

* See page 260.

240

that all of us who are gathered together here,—whether as eurythmists who already know the fundamentals of eurythmy, as beginners, or indeed as those merely interested in eurythmy,—that all of us here will feel ourselves as the helpers and promoters of eurythmy, of this art which springs from no humble source, but has as its lofty origin, that cosmic knowledge which creates from out of the spirit. If we feel ourselves as the helpers of eurythmy, either in an active or in a more passive sense, then eurythmy will be able to fulfil the mission which it can and should fulfil in the general development of Anthroposophy.

When people will see in beauty the spirit working in human movement, then this will make some contribution to the whole attitude which humanity, through Anthroposophy, should take up towards the spirit.

Let us think of all the many things which have grown up out of anthroposophical soil, forming together one great whole; and then, inspired by the Anthroposophy in our hearts, let us build up and develop each separate activity as it should and will be developed if we prove ourselves worthy of the real aims of Anthroposophy. This course of eurythmy lectures may perhaps have done something towards this end.

FOREWORD TO 1927 EDITION

It has been a task of special difficulty to weld into book form these lectures which originally depended so much upon the living co-operation of lecturer and demonstrators. These lectures were not meant as an encyclopedic recapitulation of the whole sphere of eurythmy; they were given just at that point in the evolution of eurythmy where it became necessary to review all that had been accomplished during the course of many years' activity, and which had already been carried out into the world by the various teachers. The intention was to examine and correct the results of this work and ' to gather together a number of guiding lines, developed entirely from out of the nature of eurythmy itself.' Rudolf Steiner says in the last lecture of this course that his intention was to give his lectures such a form that they would show ' how eurythmy arises out of the feeling life, out of the soul; how a eurythmic technique must be won from out of the love of eurythmy, just as everything must in reality arise out of love.' And indeed his own words streamed forth from a fountain of love, bringing help and aid to the work already accomplished,—the work which from then on was to be based on an even surer foundation. Up to this time there had been no shorthand reports of the teaching by means of which Rudolf Steiner introduced this art to the world. In the year 1912 he gave ten lessons to a seventeen year old girl, who, through the death of her father, was faced with the necessity of assisting in the maintenance of her younger brothers and sisters. She greatly wished to devote herself to some art of movement which was not based upon the materialistic tendencies of the age. This concrete fact proved the impulse for that teaching which has resulted in eurythmy. I was invited to take part in these lessons; they consisted in the rudiments of sound-formation, and a number of exercises in reality belonging to the educational aspect of eurythmy,—that is to say the basic principles of standing, walking and running, certain postures and gestures, and a number of staff-exercises and rhythmic exercises. From these basic principles several girls, pupils of the first eurythmist, worked out the educational aspect of eurythmy; later they passed on to the expression of poems by means of movements corresponding to the sounds. This was the first phase of eurythmic development. Every now and again, when the work was shown to him, Rudolf Steiner explained and corrected, answering any questions put to him. A second phase of eurythmic development began when this new art found a foothold in Dornach, at the Goetheanum. The first group of young teachers requested and received a further course, in which more especially teaching about the formation of words, word-relationships, the nature of speech, the structure of poetry was given, as also new group forms. The work was carried out into the world, but the war soon checked its activity. In order to save this art and to rescue the eurythmists from their enforced inactivity, it became necessary for me to take the work in hand. Destiny brought this task to me quite naturally, for a new style of recitation was necessary for eurythmy, and I had to find my way into this new method, to understand and develop it. I recognized the great significance of eurythmy as a regenerating source for all branches of art, and deeply regretted the fact that the eager work of these young eurythmists should be rendered fruitless by the war. There is no better remedy against the errors of taste of the present day than this new art, which leads us back to the primeval forces, to the creative forces of the universe. It is of untold benefit to mankind. Thus I worked half of the year in Germany with one group of eurythmists, and the other half of the year at the Goetheanum in Dornach, always supported and assisted by Rudolf Steiner, to whom we could turn with all our questions. The instruction we received from him in the course of time has been gathered together in book form by Annemarie Dubach-Donath, one of our best and most experienced eurythmists, the second in that line of young girls who devoted themselves to the study of eurythmy. This book, entitled *The Basic Principles of Eurythmy*, and published by the Philosophisch-Anthroposophischer Verlag, sets forth and explains these principles, thus building a foundation which is absolutely necessary if eurythmy is to be understood, and without which it would always remain incomplete.

We met together to take part in this course as if uniting in a common festival. Many were the questions put to Rudolf Steiner; he recapitulated the teaching, clearing up many things about which we held differing opinions. The whole nature of this course was that of spontaneous improvisation; diagrams were rapidly sketched on the board, exercises demonstrating certain points were carried out by the eurythmists; everything bore the character of intimate conversation and co-operative work, not of pedantic instruction. This was often the case with the teaching given by Rudolf Steiner to his pupils, but never to such a degree as in this course on eurythmy. He himself, in all probability, wished the content of these lectures first to be assimilated and experienced, and then later on cast into another form and given to the world through the agency of some other person. Now, however, when he has gone from us, his own words are what we value most. Even here,—when the effect cannot be other than fragmentary, constantly interrupted as the lectures were by practical example and demonstration,—many subtle relationships are brought to light, and we are moved to the heights and depths of our being in a way which would be impossible through the words of another. During his lectures, as he himself delivered them, the cadences of his voice seemed to stream out from spiritual depths, revealing radiant glimpses of cosmic mysteries. And now, even after his death, he still makes for us that sacrifice which he had to make throughout his whole life,—the sacrifice, that is to say, of allowing the disjointed fragments of his spirit to be preserved and written down by another hand. Those who drew life from his spirit demanded this sacrifice. None knew what it cost him. But the sacrifice was made. It has saved for our age the wisdom which reveals the relationship of universe and man; it has preserved for present-day humanity,—no longer able to remember the word of the spirit without the aid of the written record,—that store of knowledge which can raise man ever more and more to the consciousness of the concrete reality of the spirit; it contains the kindling, life-awakening spark.

Among the many branches of the spiritual work of Rudolf Steiner eurythmy was one of those which he held most dear. It developed quite organically from the smallest beginnings, adding shoot to shoot, and reaching goodly proportions, thanks to the health-giving nurture and tireless labours of its creator. It ennobled those who gave themselves to its study, compelling them more and more to put aside all that is personal; it left no room for caprice. Its inherent laws were rooted in a spiritual necessity; these laws were gladly acknowledged, for in them one experienced necessity, one experienced God. This is why eurythmy was able to arouse such heartfelt enthusiasm; many eager students banded themselves together in selfless work, so that the field of activity grew ever wider and wider. Side by side with the development of recitation, eurythmy entered into the realm of music and in this domain also it opened up fresh channels and gave fresh possibilities of expression. A new art of stage lighting came into being, following the laws of eurythmy, and a new style of dress, simpler, more impersonal, more dignified; these were based upon the experience of the colours, upon what might be called a eurythmy of colour. In its connection with the drama, eurythmy led to a means of representing those beings which otherwise had to be represented in a more or less materialistic way. The portrayal of the super-sensible and sub-sensible in earthly life now became possible. Thus, as the years went by, we were able to produce on the stage of the Schreinerei at the Goetheanum all those scenes in Faust in which the super-sensible plays a part and which otherwise are either omitted or mishandled. The romantic *Walpurgisnacht* revealed undreamed of life and intricacy of detail, and the classical *Walpurgisnacht* also, with

245

its manifold ghostly happenings. Elves, angels, the hosts of heavenly beings were represented in these performances with simplicity and dignity, and in a way entirely convincing. The greater our activity and work the greater was our gain. Every effort which resulted in deeds was rewarded by fresh gifts from our generous teacher. So many possibilities of work arose that we could not keep pace with them in the time at our disposal.

After several years of tireless training and a good deal of stage experience before friendly audiences, the time came for eurythmy to be carried out into the world. The result was striking; it was received with enthusiastic appreciation or violent opposition,—never with indifference. We were threatened with the ostracism of the cultured world; the press representatives were usually instructed to write from an antagonistic point of view, even if, as they often asserted, they themselves were enthusiastic. Representatives of other branches of art were often deeply impressed, often, also, aggressively ironical. Members of such societies as aim at reforms of all kinds felt their nebulous systems threatened by an unknown but assured and powerful force. Unprejudiced onlookers thanked God that there could be so true and pure an art. Children frequently asked if those were the angels of whom they had been told, and loud ' ohs ' and ' ahs ' of wonderment were often the eloquent testimony of their impressions. This art worked into the quagmire of our modern civilization as a purifying light or flame; the lovers of darkness gave vent to their opprobrium,—those who wished to rise up out of the low-lying levels of our civilization felt as if cleansed and purified. The power of the spirit manifested itself in this art and its effect was purifying and invigorating.

It so chances that I am writing these words in England. The life of London, the capital of the world, has been working upon me, the quintessence of that element in our modern civilization which has produced the predominance of all that is physical in life, of all that can serve our material well-being. The business life of this world-centre, its industrial and com-

246

mercial life, rushes noisily on its way. That to-day is a matter of course. But the menace to humanity is this: everywhere one hears the shrill sound of the wireless, the rasping of the gramophone, the whirring of the film; machinery has conquered on all sides, even in the realm of art; the most vital impulses are liable to waver and become mechanized. A performance which I witnessed in the Rudolf Steiner Hall in London, with its beautiful stage, a performance consisting of the interpretation of the music of early composers played on old instruments, had the effect of pictures from a past age. The performers (who were not Anthroposophists), attired in costumes of the period, produced a reposeful music full of feeling and inwardness, a music demanding leisure, which is not to be hurried, which deepens the contemplative life. The effect of such music is somewhat antiquated; but if one can persuade one's modern nerves to adapt themselves to an earlier attitude, curbing their restlessness, it has a beneficent influence. It has about as much resemblance to the hustle of modern music as the long, flowing dresses of earlier times, still admired by painters, have to the lanky legs of to-day, where the hem of the dress comes well above the knee. The effect of these legs on the stage, when looked at from the stalls of a theatre, is terribly obtrusive. They are shown off with determination; they are meant to be seen. The qualities formerly regarded as feminine and charming are but little in evidence in a modern drawing-room. An actress, if playing the part of a young girl, likes to loll about on some padded sofa; she thrusts out her legs, crossed over each other, and beyond that one has in perspective a little bobbed or shingled head. When one is faced with a whole row of such attitudes, the aesthetic elements must really be said to be lacking!

But this in only lack of beauty. What is still worse is that the very speech and gesture has been affected by this mechanical, noisy music, which rattles from all the gramophones, from the wireless, from the pianolas, and which even in many of the best London theatres has taken the place of the orchestra. They carry on their ceaseless noise during the intervals, drumming their hard sounds into the head and deadening the consciousness of the ego. When, at the end of a performance the conventional phrase of ' God save the King ' is played and the audience rises to its feet, without the slightest pause the music falls into some wild jazz. Where is the need of breathing space or a moment's consideration? —the machine needs no such thing. But the lack of any transition between two contrasted moods has a stultifying effect upon the soul. Young girls enter the stage, or drawing-room, even in Paris, with that rolling movement of hips and shoulders which negro dances have made second nature. They themselves do not notice this eternal rolling movement of the limbs: the effect is almost that of a wound-up doll, or of hypnosis. In woods, on the sea-shore, everywhere one is horrified by the sound of the gramophone and the sight of partners indulging in this sliding, rolling motion. Dancing, which seemed to be dying out when the decorative, elegant French dances lost their charm, when even the waltz and the polka had failed to interest, has come to life again in the crude and primitive form of imitated negro dances. ' We like the rhythm' several girls replied, when I inquired what was so fascinating about these dances.—But this rhythm is in reality no rhythm. It is anti-rhythmic, it is an earth force which whirls upwards, an over-emphasized or furtive and indistinct beat, an increased blood pulsation coupled with lowered consciousness. One only needs to look at the figures of the dancers, with their vacant, expressionless faces, to be convinced that this is so,—especially so with the men, who now, young and old alike, have suddenly developed a passion for dancing. These dances appeal to the lower instincts, and for this reason they have as adherents even the most blasé, and those whose souls have become lifeless and barren. But that which was merely animal nature in the case of the negro has with us become mechanical. The demons of machinery here find means of access; they gain a hold on the human being through his movement, through his vitality. They do not only influence his brain, but enter into this externalizing of that which should remain

248

as inner mood of the soul. The mechanical musical instruments exercise their powerful, soul-deadening forces, doing away with all atmosphere and feeling. And this non-rhythmic, mechanical element is even reflected in the manner of speech of modern actors on the stage. The sentences are shot out in a way which is jerky, rough and disjointed; they seem scarcely to belong to the human being, but only to his bony structure. The human being is not himself active, but is only an automaton functioning through intellect and senses. When, added to this, there is nervous, hysterical emotion, the producer's requirements may be said to be fulfilled. All this works its way into the souls of our young people, making them barren and empty. What will be the result? What is the outlook for future generations if no reaction sets in? A London newspaper is lying before me; a picture attracts my attention. The picture, entitled 'Urchin Humanity' depicts a street arab,—cheeky, impertinent, with an old face,—drawing a cart. In the centre of this cart sits Science, holding a gun: Poison Gas. On one side is the figure of Literature, eagerly perusing a book: Detective Romances; on the other side the figure of Art,—she is holding the apparatus for producing films; and below her sits Music, with a gramophone on her knee.—This is our age. Self-knowledge is shown by such a picture, and self-realization,—the only path which can lead to salvation.

One might despair; one might give way to the most drastic Spenglerism, if, in this time of need, the means of salvation had not also been given. Salvation lies in the spiritual work of Rudolf Steiner. He sounded the awakening call which can free humanity from the dangers of becoming animalized, stupified and mechanized.

That which once, in the ancient Mysteries, was offered to men as *Wegzehrung* (Sustenance by the Way), as they traversed the path leading to the unfolding of the personality, is now offered to them anew. It is offered at this moment when the personality might be annulled, when that which is human threatens to sink to the level of the sub-human if this gift is not grasped and assimilated in its very essence. The intellect alone cannot aid us here; understanding, left to itself, has led us to Agnosticism, to ' Ignoramibus ', to ' Spenglerism '. But if man opens himself to that which is spiritual, if he allows the spiritual to reveal to him his path, the creative forces of the spirit will conquer the seeds of death and transmute those forces of destruction which are now at work in ' urchin humanity '.

In order to see that which is of really great dimensions one must wait for the discovery of a new apparatus; otherwise it can as little be observed as that which is minute can be observed without the aid of the microscope. The distances of time alone may sometimes give the necessary perspective. The work of Rudolf Steiner towers so immeasurably over what may be grasped and understood at the present day that it is only the moving passage of time, with its widened outlook, which will first make possible a true valuation. It is our duty to apply ourselves to the many and various branches of the work, gradually bringing them into the range of vision; for here, on all sides may be found the life-belts to which we may cling in the surrounding waters of destruction and disintegration.

That which is seemingly limited often proves to be of the greatest significance. Let us begin with education by means of and in art; let us trace the path leading back to the source from which art had its first beginning. Truly this origin was no mean one. It was the dance of the stars and its reflection in the human sphere that was known as the dance of the planets, as Temple Dancing. Here the creative forces streamed into the human body, building its form, directing it in space, and conjuring up those forces which give to man the possibility of working creatively upon himself.

And out of these forces there arose in man the faculty of leading his inner activity over into works of art, plastic and musical. Such works of art were channels which allowed the divine to radiate down into matter. They were a reflection of the cosmos.

But when the onslaught of materialism silenced the divine forces within man, rendering them powerless, when the

250

human brain became the coffin for dead thinking and was no longer able to grasp the spiritual, then arose a deliverer. He spiritualized the intellect; he freed it from its rigidity; he restored to it its living mobility.

Indeed he brought movement into all domains of human activity. We, however, had no recollection of movement in a spiritual sense, for the movement of matter, which we had laid hold of and mastered, sufficed us, intoxicating us with its rapid motion. We did not notice that the spiritual part of our being was left passive, and that as a substitute we were intoxicating ourselves with the specific movements of sport. By this means also we alienated ourselves ever further from the spiritual impulse of movement.

We must retrace our steps with awakened consciousness; we must observe for ourselves the mighty forces of movement and whither they tend to lead us; then we shall perceive a gathering together of creative activity, the forces of which give form to the organs, and we shall gain the possibility of developing new spiritual organs in ourselves.

In this way we shall conquer the rigidity, the lifelessness, the barrenness, which to-day lead people even of the finest intelligence to the extremes of pessimism.

Once more chance has put a paper into my hand,—in Hanover, where I am writing the conclusion of this foreword. Here one may read: 'Culture (Kultur), so long as it is strong and full of motive power, works unconsciously. We are compelled to absorb and cultivate a conscious civilization. Is not this from the very outset the signal of an incurable and sterile weakness? Is it not the destruction of that seed from which springs all creative force, so that at most one may only expect a feeble echo of that which may truly be called culture? Is the circle of real culture already completed, so that there only remains for us a civilized mechanism, with perhaps some romantic glimmer remaining from the fullness of light of better days,—which also may soon fade into nothingness?' (from the *Niedersachsenbuch*, 1927).

In earlier times the inhabitants of Lower Saxony unconsciously followed a spiritual guidance, and they conquered the land of the Celtic Breton and the Gael.—As Englishmen theirs was the task of developing the consciousness soul, in so far as this is bound up with the actual personality and with physical, earthly surroundings. If the German people could raise the forces of consciousness up into the sphere of the divine ego in man, then they would have fulfilled the task of the German civilization. Then they would give to the world a new culture for which all humanity would render thanks,— whereas people turn from them, when untrue to their mission they imitate the mechanistic civilization, carrying this to its furthest extremes.

The greatest herald of the spirit of Germany proclaimed this to the German people with warning voice ever and again during the catastrophe of the world war, and he uttered these stirring words:

> Der deutsche Geist hat nicht vollendet,
> Was er im Weltenwerden schaffen soll.
> Er lebt in Zukunftssorgen hoffnungsvoll,
> Er hofft auf Zukunftstaten lebensvoll.
> In seines Wesens Tiefen fühlt er mächtig
> Verborgenes, das noch reifend wirken muss.
> Wie darf in Feindesmacht verständnislos
> Der Wunsch nach seinem Ende sich beleben,
> So lang das Leben sich ihm offenbart
> Das ihn in Wesenstiefen schaffend hält!

(The German Spirit has not completed
Its destined gift to World-Becoming.
Hope-filled, it lives in cares which fill the future,
Life-filled, it hopes for deeds on which the future must depend
And in its deepest being feels
A hidden might which yet must work to ripeness.
Opposing powers, with lack of understanding,
Desire its end. Yet of this wish how shall there be fulfilment
So long as there is manifest that life
Which in the depths sustains creative power!)

This life must be grasped by the German. It does not, however, lie in ' keeping the race pure,' as the slogan has it. It lies in the realization of his inherent ego forces, of his divine ego forces. But the path to this leads through the realm of consciousness. The consciousness of the personality, metamorphosed and raised up to the undying ' I ', possesses creative forces; it conceals the spirit in itself and will produce, not the mere echo of past culture, but a virile culture of its own.

It may seem that I have strayed far from the subject of the book which I am introducing, and yet this path leads us back to the inner regions of the temple from which the ancient civilizations arose, at first in Word and in Art,—not unconsciously, but guided by the most exalted spirits. They will come to our aid also, at this epoch when it has become necessary for each individual Spirit-Consciousness to work towards the gradual transmutation of itself into a universal Human-Ego-Consciousness. If we allow ourselves to receive this aid, we shall be in a position to open ourselves to the spirit in every sphere of activity,—in that sphere also which this book illumines with spiritual revelation and human knowledge. Then we shall no longer need to stimulate our slackened nerves by means of decadent negro dances which are hammered into us by machinery, turning us into machines and gradually killing out our finest human qualities; but we shall gain an understanding for a noble art of movement, having its source in the spirit, an art of movement which is the reflection of the Dance of the Stars, and which makes the language of the stars sound visibly within us in purity and truth.

MARIE STEINER.

November, 1927.

HOW DOES EURYTHMY STAND WITH REGARD TO THE ARTISTIC DEVELOPMENT OF THE PRESENT DAY?

Introductory words to the Eurythmy performance given in Dornach, 26th December, 1923, on the occasion of the Foundation Meeting of the General Anthroposophical Society.

The nature of eurythmy has certainly been repeatedly discussed before the most varied groups of our friends, lately also it was presented in the most varied way in the Goetheanum,* and it is indeed unnecessary to speak at this performance, which is to be given exclusively to our friends about the essential nature of eurythmy, about the basic principles, which are known to all. Yet I should like to characterize again and again from a certain standpoint both the way in which eurythmy stands in the artistic development of the present and what its position among the arts in general is. To-day I will speak a few words about how eurythmy must in fact, as it were from its very nature, be drawn out from the being of man by a spiritual world-conception, which, in accordance with the signs of the times, is making itself felt in our present age.

We look at another art which portrays the human being—the plastic art, which portrays him in his quiescent form. Whoever approaches plastic art with a certain feeling for form, whoever experiences the human being, human characteristics, through a plastic work of art does so in the best way when he has the feeling: here the human being is silent, speaking through his quiescent form.

Now we know that in the eighteenth century Lessing wrote a paper on the limits of plastic art,—it was not called

* See Rudolf Steiner, foreword to a eurythmy performance in ' Das Goetheanum ' Year 3, No. 7.   23rd Sept., 1925.

that, but that was its content,—in which he said that sculpture should in its very nature be a manifestation of that which is at rest, of that which is silent in man,—in man as a being placed into the cosmos. So that sculpture can only express that which manifests itself as silence, as stillness, in the human being. Hence any attempt to represent the human being in movement through the medium of sculpture will undoubtedly prove to be an artistic error.

In times gone by, indeed up to the time of the Renaissance, it was a matter of course that plastic art could only represent the human being in a state of rest. For it may be said: This age, which began with ancient Greece and ended with the Renaissance, was mainly concerned with the development in the human being of the intellectual soul. With regard to the inner configuration of man's being,—the sentient soul, the mind soul and the consciousness soul,—it is the mind soul, embracing as it does all that is connected with the human mind, that holds the middle place; and the mind is in fact permeated with that quiescent feeling which also comes to expression in the quiescent human form.

We live to-day in an age in which we must advance from the feeling element in man to the will element; for fundamentally speaking it is the descent into the will element which, if consciously achieved, would enable us to-day to attain to spiritual insight.

This brings us to the point where we may turn our spiritual gaze to the human being in movement; not to the human being who, as the expression of the Cosmic Word, remained silent in order to rest in form, but to the human being as he stands in the living weaving of the Cosmic Word, bringing his organism into activity in accordance with his cosmic environment.

It is this element in man which must find expression in eurythmy. And if one is able to observe things from the point of view of the spiritual science which is suited to the humanity of to-day, one will always have the feeling that form must become fluidic. Let us look at a human hand. Its silence finds expression in its quiescent form. What then is

255

the meaning of this quiescent form when the human being as a whole is taken into consideration? Its meaning is apparent when the quiescent element of feeling is allowed to hold sway as it did hold sway from the age of the ancient Greeks to the time of the Renaissance. There is certainly great significance in such a gesture as this, in which I indicate something with my hand, then allowing it to remain in a state of rest. But it does not enable us to understand what must be realized to-day with regard to man, it does not enable us to understand the human being in his totality.

It is indeed impossible to understand the human form, when observing the human being as a whole, unless one is conscious of the fact that every motionless form in man has meaning only because it is able to pass over into definite movement. What would be the significance of the human hand if it were compelled to remain motionless. Even in its motionless state the form of the hand is such as to demand movement.

When one studies the human being with that inner mobility which is essential to the Spiritual Science of to-day, then from out of the quiescent form, *movement* reveals itself on all sides. It is not too much to say that anyone who visits a museum containing sculpture belonging to the best periods of plastic art, and who looks at the figures with the inner vision arising out of the spiritual knowledge of our time, will see these figures descend from their stands, move about the room and meet each other, becoming on all sides enfilled with movement.

And eurythmy,—now eurythmy arises naturally out of sculpture. And to learn to understand this is our task also. To-day people gifted with a certain spiritual mobility feel disturbed if obliged to look for a long time at a motionless Greek statue. They have to force themselves to do it. This can, and indeed must be done in order not to spoil the Greek statue in one's own personal fantasy. But at the same time the urge remains to bring movement into this motionless form. As a consequence there arises that moving sculpture to which we give the name of Eurythmy. Here

256

the Cosmic Word is itself, movement. In eurythmy man is no longer silent but through his movement communicates innumerable cosmic secrets.

It is indeed always the case that man communicates through his own being numberless secrets of the universe. One can, however, have yet another cosmic feeling. Anyone who has a living understanding for such descriptions of cosmic evolution as are to be found in my *Outline of Occult Science* will realize from the outset that, in the case of the human form of to-day, it is as though one had allowed an inner mobility to become dried up, to become rigid. One need only to look back to the time of the Old Moon. The human being was then in a continual state of metamorphosis. Such a definitely formed nose, such definitely formed ears as man has to-day, these did not exist at that time. The once mobile forms had to become frozen. He who with his vision can transport himself into the time of the Old Moon, to him people to-day often appear as frozen, immobile beings, incapable of metamorphosis. And what we achieve by means of eurythmy, when we make it into a visible speech, is no less than this: The bringing of movement, of fluidity, into the frozen human form.

This demands a study which must in its very nature be artistic. In this sphere everything intellectualistic is positively harmful. Eurythmy is and must remain an art.

Just consider for a moment that some such eurythmy form as you have sometimes seen here in connection with poems which really have in their experience and structure the profundity, for instance, of the poems of Steffen,—just consider that such a form would best be found when, let us say—one imagines ten or twelve people of the present day. You are certainly all individually different with regard to your external form; but one can say of every person, no matter whether he has a round or long head, a pointed or blunt nose,—one can say of every person how, in the case of a poem, he would move his etheric body. And it would certainly be interesting for one to take those sitting in a certain row and show how, in the case of a poem, each one

257

of those sitting here would move in accordance with his own form, if this came about entirely from the individual characteristics of the person in question. Here are sitting, for instance, eight people in this row. In such a case quite different eurythmy forms would arise from the human form. This would be very interesting. One would have to look at many people in order to say how the human being would move for " Und es wallet und woget und brauset und zischt ".

And then one gets the idea of how the forms are necessary. Thus eurythmy is born wholly out of the moving human form, but one must be able to take up such a standpoint that, when asked why the form for a poem is such and such, one must say: Yes, that is how it is! If anyone demands an intellectual explanation in justification of such a form, then one will feel annoyed to give it, because that is really inartistic. Eurythmy is created entirely out of feeling and can also only be understood through feeling.

Of course one must learn certain things, the letters must be learned, and so on. But after all, when you write a letter, here also you do not think about how an *i* or a *b* is written, but you write because you are able to do so. The point, then, is not how the eurythmist must learn *a*, *b*, *c* but to enjoy what comes out of it in the end.

What must develop out of eurythmy is a newly created, moving sculpture. And for this living sculpture one must of course make use of the human being himself; here one cannot use clay or marble. This leads into a realm of art which, in the profoundest sense, touches reality just where sculpture departs from it. Sculpture portrays that which is dead in the human being, or at least that which is death-like in its rigidity. Eurythmy portrays all that in the human being which is of the nature of life itself. For this reason eurythmy can call forth the feeling of how the universal cosmic life laid hold of man and placed him into earthly evolution, giving him his earthly task. There is perhaps no other art through which one

258

can experience man's relationship to the cosmos so vividly as one is able to do through the art of eurythmy. Therefore this art of eurythmy, based as it is on the etheric forces in man, had to appear just at that time a modern Spiritual Science was being sought. For it was out of this modern Spiritual Science that eurythmy had to be born.

THE POSITION OF EURYTHMY IN THE ANTHROPOSOPHCIAL SOCIETY

From the 'News Sheet' (Nachrichtenblatt)
Year I. No. 22, June 8th, 1924

During the time from the middle of May to the middle of June, Frau Marie Steiner with the eurythmists from the Goetheanum is undertaking a eurythmy tour through the towns of Ulm, Nürnberg, Eisenach, Erfurt, Naumberg, Hildesheim, Hanover, Halle and Breslau. The accounts of this journey, which I receive here in the Goetheanum, speak of a profound interest which the comparatively large audiences take in the art which has arisen out of the anthroposophical movement.

That here and there a few noisy disturbers bring discord into the otherwise very gratifying reception cannot alienate him who knows the obstacles which must always, in every sphere of life, be contended with when that to which people are accustomed is faced by something new.

One would like to expect from the Anthroposophical Society that it should bring its full inner support towards the endeavours which are active in the art of eurythmy. For only with such inner support can the warmth be sustained which is necessary for those who dedicate themselves to these endeavours.

It is not everywhere known within the Anthroposophical Society upon what foundations such endeavours are built up. At the Goetheanum, under the direction of Marie Steiner, constant work is going on in order to carry out all the practices necessary before the performances. In all this work great devotion is indispensable from all those taking part. And from outside it is not always apparent how wearing it is, in artistic work, to make tiring journeys from town to town, how fretting to unfold the artistic mood during these fatiguing journeys. To succeed in carrying out such endeavours in the available circumstances certainly needs much devotion and a true enthusiasm for the cause.

Eurythmy as an art is the fruit of the spiritual impulse working in the anthroposophical movement. That which lives in the human organisation as soul and spirit comes to visible manifestation through eurythmy. Its effect upon those watching it depends upon the inner perception that in the externally visible movements of people and groups of people soul and spirit visibly unfold themselves. He only who has the artistic conception of what lies in the audible word can unfold the right sense for how the audible can, in eurythmy, be transformed into the visible. One has, as it were, the human soul-being before one's eyes.

And into this evident revelation of the human soul-being resound the arts of recitation and of music. It can be said that the art of recitation experiences in the strivings of eurythmy the essential conditions of its being. Recitation is, of course, connected in the first place with the word. But the word easily succumbs to the temptation to stray away from the artistic. It tends to become the *content* of understanding and feeling. It is, however, only the *formation* of this content which can have artistic effect. When recitation appears at the side of the eurythmic art of movement it has to unfold its formative character in full purity. It must reveal what can work formatively and musically in language. Necessary for eurythmy, therefore, was the development of the art of recitation, as this has been made possible by the devotion of Marie Steiner to this part of the anthroposophical movement. Within the Anthroposophical Society one should follow up what has arisen since the time when Marie Steiner, with a few eurythmists, began the work in 1914 in Berlin. Eurythmy could only unfold itself as a visible art of speech side by side with the artistically conceived audible art of speech. He only who has the artistic conception of what lies in the audible word can unfold the right sense for how the audible can, in eurythmy, be transformed into the visible. From the side of the public that only can be of interest which shows artistic merit. For the members of the Anthroposophical Society the point is intimately to share in the *becoming* of such a striving. For this is a part of the anthroposophical life.

In such a sharing the noblest human elements will be able to develop. And in such a development lies indeed one of the grandest tasks of the Anthroposophical Society.

Our musicians who place their artistic gifts at the service of eurythmy are bringing, I am convinced—through the way in which they do this and through the great enthusiasm which ensouls them in their work with the related art—they are bringing music forward in a quite special direction. I believe, indeed that the musical sense which lives in them finds its true *liberation* when placed in this connection. In any case, in the work of our musicians within the framework of eurythmy activity there is a deeply satisfying expansion of the musical into the general sphere of art. And its fruitfulness is shown again by the beautiful working-back upon the specifically musical.

From Marie Steiner's efforts in the sphere of eurythmy there has arisen the Eurythmeum in Stuttgart. This is based upon the idea of a eurythmy conservatorium. Eurythmy in all its branches is taught there, lectures being also given in such auxiliary subjects as poetry, aesthetics, history of art, music theory, etc. All this in accordance with that artistic conception in the light of which eurythmy must stand. What has arisen in this way in Stuttgart carries within itself many possibilities of further upbuilding.

It is deeply satisfying to see how many members from the circle of our society devote themselves with the warmest participation to the furtherance of eurythmy endeavours. This participation is in process of growing in a gratifying way. Through this there has entered into our movement a feature which is entirely consistent with the fundamental conditions of its life. For art stands midway 'between the revelations of the sense-world and spiritual reality. It is the aim of anthroposophy to place the spiritual world before mankind. Art is the reflection of the spirit in the sense-world. If art did not grow upon anthroposophical soil this could only result from some lack in this soil itself. In anthroposophical circles insight into this has been steadily increasing; it is to be hoped that such understanding will ripen more and more.

Dornach, 4 *August*, 1922

To-day I should like to give you some indications about our art of eurythmy.

We must realise that every art is limited in its sphere of work by the means of artistic expression which stand at its disposal. And an art only gains a true life of its own when, in its struggle towards achievement, it makes use simply and solely of those means of artistic expression which lie within its own sphere.

Let us take as an example the art of sculpture. The plastic art, the art of sculpture uses as its means of expression form, surface; and it must, when for instance it represents an animal form or a human form, take as its basis the fact that everything which is bound up with the human being or the animal has to be expressed by means of the modelled surface, and must consequently be carried out by the specialized technique of the same.

Let us suppose, then, that we wish to represent a smooth-coated animal. In such a case we should have to handle the marble, the bronze or the wood, in a manner quite different from that which we should have to employ if we wished to represent a rough-coated animal. We are always compelled, through these artistic means, to bring something to expression which does not actually lie within their sphere. Thus, for example, in the art of sculpture, we are obliged to use the way in which we treat the surface of our material as our means of representing that which is present in the human being himself as colour, as the natural flesh-colour. For this reason it would be wrong if, instead of modelling a statue, one tried in some way to represent the human being by means of a plaster cast. This might indeed, as far as the form is concerned, be in complete accordance with the human being, but it would only be reproducing the naturalistic human form. Such a reproduction could never give the impression of the actual human being. For in the case of the actual human being the effect is produced in the first place by means of the colour of his flesh, by his colour,—it is produced by many other things as well, for instance by his expression. All this cannot be brought into the art of sculpture. We must, therefore, give to the surface a moulding and shaping which is different from the naturalistic human form if we wish to produce an impression of the human being as a whole.

In the art of painting, for example, we again have to do with a working upon a surface. And here, in the figures we are representing, we must express by means of the treatment of colour all that is expressed in actual reality by means of form. In recent times this artistic insight has been in a measure lost, and, because people really have not understood how to confine their work in any particular art to the limits of its means of expression, the naturalistic element has crept into art to an ever greater degree. And this naturalistic principle, because it is confined in any art to a limited means of expression, brings in its train something which is inartistic and lifeless.

When, for instance, we are considering the stage, we must realize that a scene taking place on the stage and representing some aspect of life must necessarily be something quite different from the same scene taking place in ordinary naturalistic circumstances. The stage may be said to throw life up into relief, and, in arranging everything to do with the stage, we must always reckon with this fact. We must, for example, know what is signified when an actor moves from the back of the stage towards the front. On the stage this has a significance which is indeed quite different from what it would have if anyone moved in a room from the back towards the front. We must take the whole milieu into account; we must reckon with the auditorium. For a dramatic work of art unfolds itself in an interplay between

265

that which is taking place on the stage and in the auditorium.

Suppose, for instance, that in a drama one of the actors has to speak a passage which, according to its content, is intended to produce the effect of something specially intimate. This effect of intimacy could never be produced by the actor moving backwards, but the effect of intimacy is conveyed when the actor moves forward towards the front of the stage. Generally speaking, everything on the stage has a significance other than in daily life. When an actor moves from the right side of the stage (as seen from the auditorium) towards the centre, this means something entirely different from what it would be if he moved towards the centre from the left side.

We must master the means at our disposal in the sphere of dramatic art. We must reckon with the movement of the actor in this or that direction of the stage. It is not without importance when we say to ourselves: What should be done by someone wishing to express a feeling of intimacy? In naturalistic art people as a rule would merely be of the opinion that the actor should be made to catch his breath. But this, in certain cases would not produce such an effect upon the naive onlooker as would the simple method of making the actor take three, four or five steps forwards.

Let us take another art,—one which in our present age is least of any rightly understood; let us take the art of recitation and declamation. When people's attitude towards recitation and declamation is such that they believe that everything should be spoken in as naturalistic a way as possible, that all emphasis should be as naturalistic as possible, then the result is indeed inartistic. The art of declamation and recitation depends upon something quite different; here the whole point is that one knows how to study, asking: What is the character of the vowels, what the character of the consonants, what the special mood which lies in the vowel e or the vowel a? How is the pure a-mood affected by m? How is the pure a-mood affected by l? And further one must understand how such moods as lie in the vowels or consonants may spread their colour over a whole line;

266

one might perhaps extend such a mood over a whole monologue, speaking of one monologue as being recited in the *e*-mood, of another in the *a*-mood,—that is to say, one can develop the whole atmosphere and mood of some special sound, of *a* or *e*, of *m* or *l*.

Thus it is absolutely possible to develop from out of the special means at our disposal in any situation an artistic method of treatment, which does indeed define the art in question. Apart from this the point is in recitation and declamation to realise the essential difference between the epic, the lyric and the dramatic mood. And further, just in this art, quite special attention must be paid to the naïve impressions of the onlooker,—besides doing everything possible to develop the artistic feeling of whoever has to recite or declaim. This could never be achieved by naturalistic methods; it can only be achieved when one understands how to give shape and form,—the right shape and form,—not only to single sounds, but also to sentences, and even to whole passages. This is why I have repeatedly said that in the accompaniment of eurythmy by recitation and declamation the important thing is always to bring out the musical and imaginative element lying in the poet's treatment of the language. That which in ordinary naturalistic life is attained by means of emphasis must here be attained by means of the whole forming and shaping of the speech itself.

Now when we look at eurythmy from this standpoint,—in so far as it is the aim of eurythmy to be a true art,—we must ask ourselves: What are its artistic means?—You have certainly all attended performances of eurythmy, and consequently you will know that here, in the first place, we have to do with a movement of the human limbs, of the hands and arms more especially,—but also, at least in indication, with a movement of the whole human body. This is the means of expression for eurythmy as an art.

Thus it is the *movement itself* which we have to consider in the first place. And the onlooker first gains a really satisfying impression of eurythmy when he is able to perceive something in the movement as such, in the movement, for example, which belongs to a vowel or a consonant,—that is to say, in the plastic form which appears as a consequence of the movement. This is of the first importance. But also we should not forget that eurythmy really is an actual visible speech, and as such it is an expression of the soul, just as is the speech which manifests in sound. So that everything which is to be represented in eurythmy must depend solely upon such means as can produce upon the eye just such an effect as the language of sound produces on and through the ear.

Thus it would be quite wrong if anyone were to think that ordinary mime or play of feature can have any significance in eurythmy. This play of feature, this use of facial expression is quite without significance; only that has significance which really belongs within the sphere of movement. The onlooker must, then, be able absolutely to forget, in the essence of the movement, anything which depends upon mime or any other use of the face, or upon the face itself. Speaking in an ideal sense either beauty or lack of beauty in the face of the eurythmist is quite without importance. The attention must be absolutely concentrated upon the movement itself.

But in its movement eurythmy is itself a language; it is the expression of the human soul. And no one,—let us speak for example of a sculptor or an actor,—would be able to give form to a sound or a combination of sounds, or be able to give shape to a surface, if he did not possess feeling, the feeling for the curved surface or for the structure and formation of sounds. It is not so much a question of the performer, just at the moment of performance, having a feeling for what ought to be called up in the audience or for how it should be called up (for this would only lead him into error) but the point is actually to feel the *structure of the sounds the shape and form of the sounds*. The sculptor too must have a *feeling for his surface*. The sculptor has a different feeling according to whether he feels a round or a flat surface. This is not a feeling that one wishes to display;

it is the artistic feeling which is developed by the artist within the sphere of his means of artistic expression.

The eurythmist also can develop such a feeling. And, in a performance of eurythmy, it is only when the right feeling, the right inner attitude towards the movements is present, that a real effect upon the soul of the onlooker is achieved.

Let us realize for once what this can mean. Let us take some movement,—any sound, which would make the eurythmist move the hand and arm in this way, and then hold it for a moment (demonstrating the movement);— here we have the *movement* or the plastic posture into which the movement has led us over.

Now the effect of this movement will only be ensouled when the eurythmist, apart from making the movement, actually feels in the movement itself the sensation, here in this upward direction, of something of the nature of tangible air. The sensation must be somewhat different from that of ordinary air; it is as if we had to do with air which is perceptible, tangible; it is as if something were twined around the arm, something we had to carry. We may think of this as the *feeling;* the arm is moved in such and such a way and the feeling ensues; the eurythmist feels something touching the arm quite lightly, a slight pressure, even a slight tension. If we represent this in somewhat expressionistic form, we may say that here, as it were, we fashion a veil. And the onlooker sees, when the eurythmist really uses the veil with skill, all this expressed in the veil. The veil is arranged so that the eurythmist feels a slight pressure here, a slight tension there; and then the onlooker *sees* what the eurythmist *feels.* It is possible in the movements of eurythmy to pour one's whole feeling into the forms taken by the veil.

This is, of course, speaking of the matter from a very idealistic point of view, for such things cannot be achieved all at once; they should, however, at least form a goal towards which the eurythmist must gradually strive. This is why the addition of veils to our performances of eurythmy

269

was completely justified. For the veil is, in its very nature, of real assistance to the onlooker, helping him to see in the external plastic movement what the fluidic feeling inherent in the movements of eurythmy is. And again, when we have such a working together of *movement* and *feeling* as I have described, then already we have represented some part of the soul life. For in the place of thought we have movement, and we contact the feeling quite directly. Further, something of very real assistance to the onlookers would be brought about if the colour of the veil were to have some special relationship to the colour of the dress; for it is in the dress that the movement is really brought to expression, while feeling is made visible by the veil.

Thus we are able to present, in beautiful expressionistic form this interplay between movement and feeling. And one may say that if, for instance, the dress is of a colour which corresponds in some measure to the *e*-sound,—when the dress is of some special colour,—then the veil must be of another colour. These two colours must, however, stand in a relationship towards each other corresponding to the relationship between movement and feeling.

Of course, in an actual performance of eurythmy, this cannot be carried out exactly, for it is obviously impossible to change dress and veil for each separate sound. I have already pointed out, however, that we may, if we penetrate with artistic feeling right into the essence of the whole matter, speak of certain moods; we may speak of an *e*-mood or an *u*-mood, and it is possible to carry this over, not merely into lines and verses, but into a whole poem. And when we have a feeling for the fact: This poem is written in the mood of *i*, and that poem in the mood of *e;*—or when, let us say, we are able to feel: In this poem when, having two eurythmists, we arrange that one expresses the character of the *e*-mood by means of dress and veil and the other the character of the *i;*—then once again we are able to bring to a somewhat more complicated expression, in the interplay of these two moods, the actual mood of the poem.

Such experiments in the harmonizing of dress and veil

have, of course, already been attempted in poems as a whole; for it is these things which must form the basis of our work. But they cannot be said to rest upon mere nebulous fantasy; they must be experienced with inner artistic feeling, they must be studied artistically. Only then can they be represented with such reality and truth that the onlooker, even if completely ignorant of the whole matter, will nevertheless have, albeit in quite a naïve way, the corresponding impression.

Now, however, in a performance of eurythmy we must consider yet a third element. This is the element of will, the *character*. If you take some sound and picture how it should be represented in eurythmy, you will say to yourselves: In the movement, in the first place, we have represented something which is similar to the whole treatment and formation of speech in recitation. The whole way in which speech is treated, whether pictorial or musical, is expressed in eurythmy by means of the movement.

The feeling which the reciter also brings into his recitation, the *feeling*, this is made really visible in what the eurythmist himself must experience in his own fantasy. It is as if there were here a slight feeling of pressure, there of tension,—and this has a great effect upon the movements; quite naturally, quite instinctively, the movements themselves become different with the differing feelings of the eurythmist. This is what permeates the whole thing with life and soul. And it is good when the eurythmist is not merely master of the external movement as such, but when this feeling also is present. In the forming of an *e*, for instance, one does, quite definitely, have a slight sensation in some place or another; and it is good when one is able, in imagination, to give oneself up to these slight sensations. Then the movement itself gains a soul-quality quite different from that which it has when carried out mechanically.

But the reciter also introduces into his recitation an element of will. He speaks quietly, let us say, in one place; he gains strength; often he speaks out quite loudly. This is the will-element. And this will-element,—which I should like

271

in the realm of art to name ' character ',—can also be carried over into a performance of eurythmy. Now suppose that in some sound or other you have to hold the arm in this way,—and the hand here,—(demonstrating the movement). Quite involuntarily, out of your own instinctive artistic feeling, you will create something different when you hold the hand relaxed, yielding it up to its own weight, or when you stretch it out. And just as the reciter by exerting more or less strength and power in his speech, brings character into language, so too you can bring character into eurythmy.

You will, for instance, give a different character from what you are showing by means of your arm, when, as a eurythmist you do not merely give yourself up to your fantasy, but actually bring this fantasy into outward expression. Let us say that in the case of certain letters, or in some passage which you wish to express, the forehead takes on a slight tension, or you feel in some movement that you exert a certain strength of the muscles of the upper arm, or you have the feeling, that at some point you must put down the foot quite consciously with a certain pressure on the floor;— all this forms the third element which must be brought into eurythmy, the *character*. Thus we really have the possibility of expressing the whole soul life in a performance of eurythmy.

Now you see, my dear friends, the remarkable thing is this: If one really puts into practice the thoughts which I have just set before you, then, simply by expressing eurythmy in a certain way, one creates the impulses which underlie what is being sought after to-day as a special form of art,— expressionism in art. For eurythmy is, from a certain point of view, absolutely expressionistic. Only it does not make use of the many absurd means which are made to serve so-called Expressionism; it makes use of those means whereby one can create forms of expression really artistically. It makes use of movements of the physical body, and by this means feeling is poured into the limbs, character is poured into the limbs, as I have just described.

Now in our performances, which are still, of course, only at the very beginning of their development, we have always endeavoured to carry out just these things of which I have been speaking,—to carry them out in such a way that the sounds have been treated at least according to these principles. We have endeavoured to find for each sound a justifiable means of expression, justifiable, because in the choice of one colour the *movement* is definitely represented, in a second colour the *feeling* (this is shown in the veil and is consequently only to be seen at a performance), and in a third colour the *character* is brought to expression. So that in eurythmy you are able to represent each sound by means of colour, according to *movement*, *feeling* and *character*.

In this way one may perhaps achieve a two-fold result. In the first place one may see in how far eurythmy can attain to what is artistic by its own means. For everything which is to be achieved artistically in the realm of eurythmy, limited as this is to the stage where everything has to take place,—all this may be summed up in Movement, Feeling and Character, as I have explained them here. The sculptor must achieve everything by means of his treatment of the surface, the reciter by his forming and shaping of the sounds the musician by his forming and shaping of the tones; and so also must the eurythmist achieve all that is possible to achieve by means of movement, feeling and character. What lies outside this must not be considered. This is the sphere of expression for the art of eurythmy, and by these means everything has to be achieved.

From lectures given on 4th August, 1922 (Dornach)
26th August, 1923 (Penmaenmawr).

We have recently made the attempt here at Dornach, to produce figures representing the movements of Eurythmy. And at the performances given at Oxford* we showed how an understanding of eurythmy may be helped by means of such figures, and how they may serve to clear up our ideas with regard to the nature of this art. From what I am now going to say in this connection you will see that in these figures I have at least attempted to further the understanding of eurythmy from more than one point of view.

In these figures I have been able to reproduce just those three elements of eurythmy of which I have previously spoken. It is possible by this means to increase the appreciation of the onlookers; and at the same time the eurythmists themselves may learn infinitely much from looking at these figures, because they represent those elements of eurythmy which are absolutely essential. As I am showing you these representations, I must ask you first of all to notice that they should not in any way be copied or imitated: Reproduction strictly prohibited. That is the first point. And the second is that, if I now show them to you, you will not all push forward and thus cause confusion.

We have, in the first place, tried to represent the letters of the alphabet in the way I have just described. Thus you see here, in these figures, representations of the human being from which everything not belonging to the sphere of eurythmy has been omitted. You must not expect either pictorial or plastic representations of the human form;

---

* These figures, which are carved out of wood and coloured, are made at the Goetheanum at Dornach, where they may be bought. They were shown for the first time at Oxford, during a Conference at which Rudolf Steiner gave a course of lectures on the Art of Education.

for here the human being has been depicted entirely from the point of view of eurythmy. It is, then, only the eurythmic aspect of the human being which has been taken into account; but every sound has been represented with the utmost completeness and detail. For this reason the eurythmy figures have no faces, or, to be more correct, their faces are used to express the character of the movement, the form of the movement, and so on.

Thus, taking these figures in their order, you have: A. E. I. O. U. D. B. F. G. H. That part of the figure which would usually represent the face is here formed in such a way as to represent the movement. This can, of course, only be indicated; but it is quite a good eurythmic exercise to picture oneself in fancy as really appearing like the figure in question. Proceeding, then, we have the letters: T. S. R. P. N. M. and L.

Let us, for example, take this eurythmy figure, which represents the experience lying behind the sound H. Now one might ask: In which direction is the face looking? Is it looking upwards or straight ahead?—This is really a matter of no consequence; we are concerned with something quite different. In the first place this figure, taken as a whole, represents the eurythmic movement, that is to say, the movement of the arms and of the legs. In the second place the figure shows how in the forms of the veil, in the way in which the veil is held, drawn closer, thrown into the air, allowed to fall or to undulate, the actual movement, that is to say, the more intellectual expression of the soul life in eurythmy, can be made more deeply expressive.

The significance of the different colours is always indicated on the backs of the figures. Then, in certain places, as for instance here on the head, we have the indication as to where the eurythmist, in carrying out the movement, should exert a certain tension of the muscles. Let us now examine this eurythmy figure and we shall see how the effect of the movement is made more complete by means of the treatment of the face. Observe how here, where blue is painted on the forehead, there is a tension of the muscles, as also here at the nape of the neck, while here (indicating the figure) the muscles are left more relaxed. In eurythmy one can differentiate quite exactly between the experience of moving the arm with the muscles relaxed and the experience of moving the arm with muscles that are stretched and tense, or with an exertion of the muscles in the fingers for instance. Thus, when taking up a bending posture, the feeling is quite different when the muscles involved are consciously exerted, from what it is when these muscles are allowed to relax and the back simply bends of itself. By means of this muscular tension, which must be inwardly experienced by the eurythmist, character is brought into the movement.

Thus it may be said: In the way in which the movement is formed there lies,—or rather the movement itself actually manifests,—all that the soul wishes to express by means of this visible speech. In the same way, however, as *words* have their timbre, their own special tone, brought about by the feeling lying within them, so too the *movement*,—by means of the way in which it is coloured by fear, for instance, when this is expressed in a sentence, or by joy, or delight,—so too must the movement be permeated by feeling. And this can be done by the use of the veil, by the way in which the veil is made to undulate, to float in the air, to sink down, and so on. Thus, movement accompanied by the veil is movement permeated by feeling. And movement accompanied by this inner tension of the muscles, is movement which carries with it the element of character. When a eurythmist experiences this tension or relaxation of the muscles in the right way, it can also be perceived by the onlookers. There is no necessity to explain and interpret all this, for the audience will actually feel everything that can be brought into the language of eurythmy by means of character, feeling and movement.

The figures arose through the initiative of Miss Maryon;* they have, however, been further worked out according to my indications.

Looking at the way in which these figures are carried out, both as regards the carving and the colouring, we find that

*Edith Maryon, sculptress at the Goetheanum (died 1924)

the essential thing is to separate all those elements in the human being which do not belong to the realm of eurythmy from those elements which are in themselves eurythmic. If a eurythmist were to use charm of face in order to please, this would in no way belong to eurythmy; the eurythmist must understand how to make use of the face by means of the muscular tension of which I have spoken. For this reason anyone possessing a truly artistic perception will in no way prefer a beautiful eurythmist to one who is less beautiful. In all these matters no attention need be paid to what a human being looks like, simply as a human being, apart from the movements of eurythmy; such a thing must be left entirely out of account.

Thus in the formation of these figures, we have represented only that part of the human being which may be expressed through the movements of eurythmy.

It would indeed be a very good thing if this principle were more generally applied in the development of art as a whole; for it really is necessary, in the case of any art, to separate those things which do not come within its sphere from those things which should be expressed by means of its own special medium. And in the case of eurythmy, in the case of a manifestation of the life of the human body, soul and spirit which is so direct and so true, one must be specially careful to ensure the putting aside of all those elements in the human being which do not definitely belong to the art of which we are speaking.

Thus I have always said, when asked at what age a person can do eurythmy, that there are no age limits; beginning at three until the age of ninety, the personality can fully find its place in eurythmy, for every period of life can—as in other ways also—reveal its beauties in eurythmy.

All that I have been saying is related to eurythmy in its artistic aspect, to eurythmy purely as an art. And it was indeed as an art that eurythmy first came into being. At that time, in 1912, there was as yet no thought of anything else; the aim was to bring eurythmy before the world as an art.

Then, when the Waldorf School was founded, it was

discovered that eurythmy could also be an important means of education, and we have since been able to prove that eurythmy is completely justifiable from this aspect also. In the Waldorf School eurythmy has been made a compulsory subject from the lowest to the highest class, both for boys and girls; and experience has proved that this visible speech or visible song, which is learned by the children, is acquired by them in a way which is just as natural as that in which they acquired ordinary speech and song in their earliest childhood. Children accept eurythmy as something quite self-understood. And we have also noticed that all other forms of gymnastics, when compared with eurythmy, prove themselves somewhat one-sided. For these other forms of gymnastics bear within them, as it were, the materialistic ideas of our age, and are based mainly upon the laws of the physical body. The physical body is of course also taken into account in eurythmy, but here we have a working together of body, soul and spirit; so that eurythmy may be said to be a form of gymnastics which is permeated through and through with soul and spirit. The child feels this. He feels, with every movement that he makes, that he is not forming the movements merely out of physical necessity. He feels how his life of soul and spirit flows into the movements of the arms, into the movements of the whole body. The child comprehends eurythmy in the inner depths of his soul. And now that we have a certain number of years of experience in the Waldorf School behind us, we are able to see what eurythmy is expecially able to develop. It is initiative of will, that quality so much needed by modern man, which is specially cultivated by eurythmy as a means of education. One must, however, be quite clear that, if eurythmy were only to be introduced into schools and not given its full value as an art, a complete misunderstanding would arise. Eurythmy must primarily take its place in the world as an art, just as the other arts also have their places in the world. We are taught the other arts at school when they have an independent artistic existence; and eurythmy also can be taught in the schools when, as an art, it is acknowledged and appreciated, thus becoming part of our modern civilization.

Later on a considerable number of doctors found their way into the anthroposophical movement, and through their activities the art of medicine began to be cultivated from the point of view of Anthroposophy. At this time the need made itself felt to apply the movements of eurythmy,—movements which are drawn out from the healthy human organism and in which the human being can be revealed and manifested in a way which is in truth suited to his organism,—to apply these movements in the realm of healing. Looked at from this aspect eurythmy may be said to be that part of the human being which demands free outlet. Anyone understanding the nature of a hand will know that a hand in the true sense is simply non-existent when it is regarded as something motionless. The fingers are quite without meaning when they are regarded as something motionless; their meaning first becomes apparent when they grasp at something and take hold of it, when movement arises out of the quiescent form. One can see the inherent movement in the fingers and hand. It is the same with the human being as a whole; and that which has come into being as eurythmy really is the healthy outpouring of the human organism into movement. Thus, when eurythmy is applied as curative eurythmy in the realm of therapeutics, the movements, although similar in nature, differ from those of artistic eurythmy; for they must, when used curatively, work back with a healing influence upon some particular part of the organism.

In this case, again, we have had considerable success in our treatment of the children in the Waldorf School. Naturally a real insight into child-nature is essential. Let us suppose that we are dealing with a child who is weak and ailing. He is made to do those movements which could help to bring about recovery. Results have proved,—this can be said in all modesty,—that we have here had the most brilliant success. But all these things, and everything arising out of them, can only be successful if eurythmy as an art is really brought to complete development.

A statement must here be made: we are at the beginning. We have, however, certainly progressed some little way with eurythmy, and we are seeking to develop it ever further. At first, for instance, there were no silent forms at the beginning of a poem, which represents what can be expressed as introduction and again what can be expressed as the drawing to a conclusion. At first, too, there were not the changes of lighting, which must also be so conceived that the point is not that each separate situation should be followed by one or another lighting effect; but a light eurythmy has itself come about. The essential matter is not how a certain light effect is suited to what is happening at a particular moment on the stage, but the whole eurythmy of light, the play of one lighting effect into another, which itself produced a light eurythmy,—this bears within itself the same character, the same kind of experience, which otherwise comes to expression on the stage in the movements of a single human being or a group. Thus in the development of the stage picture, in the further perfecting of eurythmy, much will have to be added to what we are now able to see.

The wooden eurythmy figures are carried out in a special way. You must not look for anything in the nature of a plastic reproduction of the human form. This belongs to the sphere of sculpture or of painting. Here, in these eurythmy figures, it is only that part of the human being that is truly eurythmic which should be represented. Thus there is no question of a beautiful plastic reproduction of the motionless human form; the point here is to reproduce that aspect of the human being which is able to express itself in movements subject to form and themselves formative.

By means of these figures, certain details of the eurythmic movements, postures and gestures can be brought out and emphasized. These figures are only intended to reproduce such eurythmic impulses as can actually be led over into movement. In each figure there is embodied a three-fold eurythmic impulse; the *movement* as such, the *feeling* lying in the movement, and the *character* which wells up from the soul and pours itself into the movement.

Dornach, 21st July 1923

The fact that eurythmy originated within the Anthroposophical Movement is not in the least arbitrary, even if the actual circumstances of the case seem almost like chance. Eurythmy developed in such a way that it was only in the course of years that its essential character was revealed. The whole process of the development of eurythmy has been such that it could only have emanated from the Anthroposophical Movement, this Movement which is suited to the needs of modern times and which is in keeping with the conditions of the present and near future.

Eurythmy must be looked upon as a quite particular art, an art which is based upon the revelation of the nature and being of man through movements of the limbs carried out by a single human being or a group of human beings, either standing still or moving in space.

I have often called this revelation of the human being ' visible speech '. It is visible speech in so far as the content of a poem or piece of music may, by its means, be brought to expression through human gesture based on laws not less exact than those which would be present if the same poem or piece of music were to be expressed through speech or song. Everything which may truly be termed art springs from a source which must be looked for in the spiritual world. It must be recognized, for instance, that architecture originated from quite definite conceptions of a supersensible nature. One may call to mind the external fact that, the further we look back in time, the more certainly do we find that monuments were erected over burial places. And when we call to mind such thoughts as are bound up with the erection of the tombstone, these thoughts would take some such form as this.

We must say to ourselves: The human being, when regarded in his entirety, does not achieve the goal of his existence by earthly life alone. He forsakes the physical body with his true being when he passes through the gate of death. His existence is continued beyond the boundary of his life on earth.

The question arises: In what way will the human being be received by the cosmos when he forsakes his physical body?—and anyone who is able to perceive as imagination this mystery of the human being, anyone able to solve this riddle imaginatively, will discover that the answer is contained in the forms of the memorial monument or tomb.

A monumental memorial stone erected over a grave is moulded in forms which seem to conceal in themselves those lines and directions along which the soul, when released from the body, will wing its way into the wide spaces of the cosmos. The tombstone answers for us the question: What are the directions taken by the soul when it forsakes the physical body?

This of course is a very radical conception of architecture. For the conception of architecture may quite justifiably be widened out so as to include certain buildings necessary for life on earth. We can then put the question to ourselves in another form, albeit this is more prosaic: If the human being, while on the earth, is obliged to have the protection of some quite definite shelter for that which is the vehicle of his soul during earthly life, what architectural surroundings suited to what he has to do on earth must he have for his physical body?

I can only touch on these things, but I wish to point out by their means how architecture, for instance, has emanated from a supersensible origin, from a spiritual vision.

And again, when examining plastic art, one will find that the origin of sculpture lies in the answer to the question: What was the work of the Gods on the human form, and what does the human being himself make out of this form during his life on earth? What in this human form is the gift of the Gods? How does the soul-life of the human being influence this divine gift?

That which is added to this divine gift by the soul-life of man is left out of account by the sculptor as not belonging to art. That which in the human form is the gift of the Gods was what was originally made manifest through plastic art.

It was during an age in which people pondered the question: What are the directions taken by the soul after death? —that monumental architecture came into existence. This may still be seen from those Catholic Churches where the altar is a tomb or memorial, and even from the Gothic churches, for these are erected over a tomb. Just as architectural conceptions were originally born out of a supersensible vision, so the conceptions of sculpture arose in an age in which people were considering the question: In what way is the human body a gift of the Gods?

In the case of each individual form of art it is possible to point out how in the corresponding epoch of time the origin of a particular form of art arose out of the raising of human consciousness into supersensible worlds. And all naturalistic tendencies in art, everything which is not a spiritual inheritance, must be looked upon as signs of decadence, as signals of the downfall of art.

From this one may see that the origin of any art can only be traced back to supersensible worlds.

When we examine the special character of our present age, it speaks to us on all sides of the way in which the forces of the subconscious and of the unconscious are weaving and working in the psycho-spiritual life of man. Most people to-day, however, allow their unconscious life to remain unconscious. Formerly, when anyone showed a certain tendency in his soul-life, people simply expressed their trust in the goodness of God, which meant that they were not going to bother any more about it. And to-day also it must be said of most people who talk about 'the unconscious', that they also allow the unconscious life to remain unconscious; they are not really troubling about it. On the other hand, it is the task of anthroposophical spiritual knowledge to raise up this unconscious life and unite it with a super-consciousness, to grasp what lives directly in the human being as psychic-spiritual in its connection with the higher spirituality.

In this respect, however, we find that, as a means of human expression, speech can be said only partially to reveal the human being. Speech is above all the vehicle of thought; and the way in which thought has developed in our modern civilization has led to the loss of poetry through too much thinking about it. This shows itself most clearly in the fact,—in spite of a healthy reaction in this direction,—that it is no longer possible to recite or declaim in a way which is really artistic. It is only with years of work and infinite pains that Frau Dr. Steiner has succeeded in leading declamation and recitation back to their true form.

A true art of recitation and declamation reveals the essential nature of poetry. For the nature of poetry may only be discovered by one who with full inner understanding can echo the words of the poet: ' Spricht die Seele, so spricht, ach, schon die Seele nicht mehr '. (If the soul speaks, then alas, the soul speaks no more.) When the soul comes to the lips, finding expression in words which have long lost their connection with the realities of the universe, then we have prose; we no longer have poetry. We only re-discover poetry when we return to a manner of speech in which the words wing their way in greater or lesser curves, in undulating waves, or lines, sharp and angular, thus forming themselves into the strophe or verse. Such pictures of the imagination as are sought by the true poet must be led over into the rhythms of the Iambic or the Trochaic, into pulse or beat, into the melodic phrase which can transform speech into music. Then we reach something which lies beyond words; whereas most people to-day emphasize the prose element in

284

recitation and declamation,—even if, as I have said, a reaction has already set in.

Speaking in a wide sense, however, we must hold to the fact that a poem can only fully be understood when the following is borne in mind.

The reciter or declaimer has no means at his disposal other than the utterance of words. All the possibilities of his art lie in the way the words are spoken. Anyone who understands how to listen to recitation or declamation with the ear of an artist feels conjured up within him an impression either imaginative or musical, a picture arising out of the actual sounds of speech, or out of the musical element in speech,— both of which are on a far higher level than thought.

Thought is a reflection of sense-impressions. We ascend to the supersensible. When we express thought by means of speech, then, because thought lives in the breath, it calls upon that which unites itself with the breath. And with the breath is connected the pulsation of the blood.

The pulsation of the blood, even to its slightest variations, expresses the experiences and perceptions of the soul; it is the expression of the soul-life. Anyone able to enter into these things with true insight is aware that, if we speak, for instance, such a word as ' Klingen ', the blood-pulsation during the first syllable ' Kling ', where there is the *i*-sound, differs from that during the second syllable, where the sound is *e*. When, with the help of the breath, thought is allowed to stream into words, the blood-pulsation, the inner movement of the human being, is stimulated.

This process continues as long as we remain in the sphere of thought. If thought clothes itself in pictures, as it can do by means of words, then we have a task different from the mere stimulation of the activity in the blood.

At the present time, when anyone speaks the sound *i*, it is spoken with the greatest indifference. It is an *i* merely, a sound which occurs in so and so many words. But this was not the case when the *i* originally appeared in human life, when it was literally wrested out of the being of man.

Anyone really able to experience the *i* would feel the way in

285

which this sound is permeated by the breath, and would also realize the intimate connection of the breath with the pulsation of the blood. He would know that with the utterance of the sound *i* the speaker places himself, his own being, as it were, in space. With the *e*-sound, on the other hand, he feels an inner spiritual experience. When he utters the sound *o* he must have the feeling: the spiritual reveals itself before him. For anyone who can feel and experience language, each individual sound transforms itself into a picture, taking on quite definite contours.

Language is rich in feeling and this manifests itself in the transition from one sound to another. In the course of civilization we have lost that inner jubilation which should be experienced in the case of certain words. Soberness and indifference have conquered and the soul-life of the human being has become soured and morose. This is why, when modern civilization speaks, one frequently feels that words are produced by tongues coated with a mixture of salt and vinegar. In this civilized manner of speaking, articulation has become such that all sounds tend towards a type of hissing dental sound; they have the effect of a mixture of salt and vinegar on the tongue. But the primal language of humanity was a liquid honey. Language is essentially sweet in its nature; and it is the means by which the being of man reveals itself in sound. Poetry to-day is fettered when it struggles to embody feeling in words, we have lost from language the feeling which it once possessed.

If this feeling is to be re-awakened, language as such must be raised to a higher level. We must realize that human speech in all its aspects is, as it were, overshadowed by a heavenly world, wherein the whole content of the soul-life of man is expressed in a mighty panorama.

When one gains the possibility of perceiving that archetype of which speech is the shadow, one becomes aware of an imaginative language in which imaginations can be expressed through the microcosm, a little world, through man, who is enabled by his form as a spatial being to bring all mysteries to expression.

286

When one has learned to know those imaginations which reveal themselves in their relationship to all the separate forms of speech, one may then pass over to the separate forms of song. And when these are translated into the sphere of human movement we get this art of eurythmy. There is an imaginative revelation of language. Language to-day has become intellectualistic. If we go back to the imaginative origin of language,—and we must do this, for in each and every sphere we must find our way back to what is spiritual,—then we shall feel how necessary it is to bring imagination into language once more. This may be done by making use, as the most significant means of artistic expression, of the possibilities of human movement in space, of the actual movements in space of the human being himself. When we wish to give expression to the deeper elements lying behind language we must do more than merely influence the circulation of the blood, which we do in speech owing to the connection existing between the breathing and the blood. We must enter a realm which soars, as it were, above the head, above thoughts, above abstract language; we must enter the realm of imaginative language. For this we need, not the circulation of the blood merely, which is influenced when we speak even when standing still; but we must pass over from the circulation of the blood into the visible movements of the human being himself. Then the gestures in the air which are produced by speech,—for we unconsciously impress the imagination into air-gestures,—are transformed into *visible gestures*. And these visible gestures are eurythmy.

Eurythmy has arisen out of the very nature of our age and out of its fundamental needs. Just as one can show how architecture had to arise out of one particular epoch, and how sculpture, painting and music arose in their corresponding epochs, so one day people will understand that eurythmy, this art of human movement, was bound to arise out of this our present age.

Complete Edition of the works of Rudolf Steiner in German, published by the Rudolf Steiner Verlag, Dornach, Switzerland, by whom all rights are reserved.

Writings

1. Works written between 1883 and 1925
2. Essays and articles written between 1882 and 1925
3. Letters, drafts, manuscripts, fragments, verses, inscriptions, meditative sayings, etc.

Lectures

1. Public Lectures
2. Lectures to Members of the Anthroposophical Society on general anthroposophical subjects.
   Lectures to Members on the history of the Anthroposophical Movement and Anthroposophical Society
3. Lectures and Courses on special branches of work:
   Art: Eurythmy, Speech and Drama, Music, Visual Arts, History of Art
   Education
   Medicine and Therapy
   Science
   Sociology and the Threefold Social Order
   Lectures given to Workmen at the Goetheanum

The total number of lectures amounts to some six thousand, shorthand reports of which are available in the case of the great majority.

Reproductions and Sketches

Paintings in water colour, drawings, coloured diagrams, Eurythmy forms, etc.

When the Edition is complete the total number of volumes, each of a considerable size, will amount to several hundreds. A full and detailed Bibliographical Survey, with subjects, dates and places where the lectures were given is available. All the volumes can be obtained from the Rudolf Steiner Press in London as well as directly from the Rudolf Steiner Verlag, Dornach, Switzerland.